IMAGES
of America

HUDSON RIVER STATE HOSPITAL

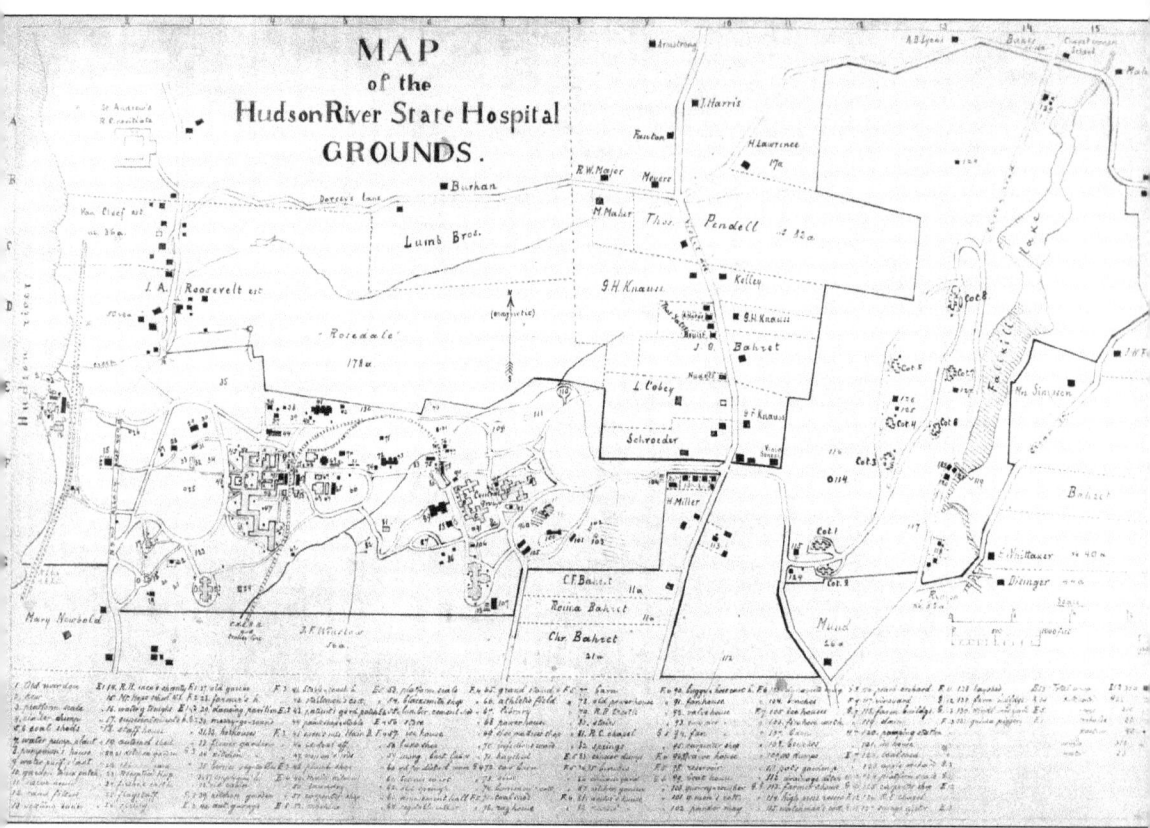

This early map of the Hudson River State Hospital displays the surrounding parcels of land belonging to private citizens. The Roosevelt Land is marked at top left. Near this marking, one can see Rosedale, where the FDR home would be constructed; it was later known as Hyde Park, New York. Drafted sometime in the late 1890s, the early structures of the hospital—consisting of the main building, the central group, and several freestanding cottages—are identifiable. (Courtesy of the Hudson River State Hospital Nurses Alumni Association.)

ON THE COVER: The most commanding view on the grounds at Hudson River was the ornate main building. This massive work of red brick and weighty stone trim does not muster feelings of ominousness, as many other public institutional structures do. A relationship of approachability is almost instantaneously established between the structure and the individual. In 1986, this building was awarded National Historic Landmark status. After 17 years of abandonment, it is scheduled to receive a second life from a developer as private living quarters. (Courtesy of the Hudson River State Hospital Nurses Alumni Association.)

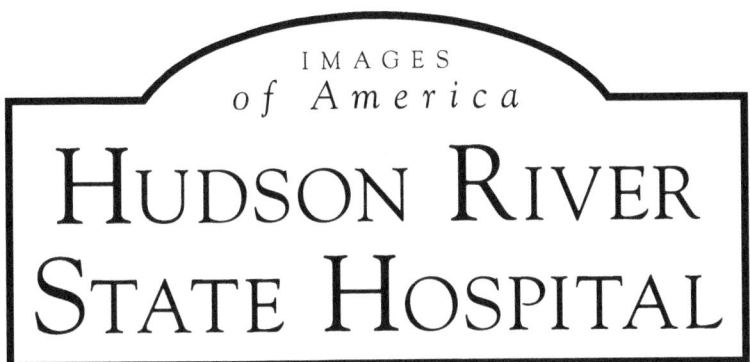

IMAGES
of America

HUDSON RIVER STATE HOSPITAL

Joseph Galante, Lynn Rightmyer, and the
Hudson River State Hospital Nurses Alumni Association

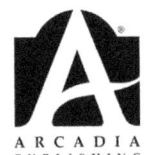

ARCADIA
PUBLISHING

Copyright © 2018 by Joseph Galante, Lynn Rightmyer, and the Hudson River State Hospital Nurses Alumni Association
ISBN 978-1-4671-2969-5

Published by Arcadia Publishing
Charleston, South Carolina

Library of Congress Control Number: 2018941676

For all general information, please contact Arcadia Publishing:
Telephone 843-853-2070
Fax 843-853-0044
E-mail sales@arcadiapublishing.com
For customer service and orders:
Toll-Free 1-888-313-2665

Visit us on the Internet at www.arcadiapublishing.com

In memory of all the staff and patients who resided at Hudson River State Hospital. May your legacy of benevolence and compassion be not forgotten.

Contents

Acknowledgments		6
Introduction		7
1.	Establishment, Construction, and Growth	11
2.	Employee Life	43
3.	Nursing and Treatment	65
4.	Fire and Police	83
5.	The Farms	95
6.	Patient Life and Activities	105
About the Hudson River State Hospital Nurses Alumni Association		127

ACKNOWLEDGMENTS

This publication would not be possible without the thousands of laborious hours hospital and governmental staff spent preserving the facility's history. A special dedication to the Hudson River State Hospital Nurses Alumni for continuingly safeguarding the rich past of this progressive hospital, as well as providing the images in this publication, is obligatory. A tremendous gratitude is owed to all former employees, especially alumni association president Margret Kidder, Linda Hacksteiner, Patricia Kickham, Patricia Toth, Len Peluso, and Lynn Rightmyer for their unwavering commitment to preserving history, even after closure of the facility. Without the support of Karen Nicholsen, New York State Office of Mental Health historic integrity officer, this publication would not have come from idea to reality. The utmost thanks go to colleague and friend Craig Williams, retired senior historian at the New York State Museum, for his wisdom, encouragement, personal time, and curatorial expertise. Both Karen's and Craig's tireless work over the past 30 years in the historic preservation of mental health history across the state inspired much of this author's work.

I was gifted with the absolute privilege to work with some of the most outstanding staff conceivable in public behavioral health. Under their tutelage, I grew from an inexperienced teenager to a man of conviction and purpose. From the depths of my heart, thank you to all the men and women in public service who invested their energy, generosity, and time in me to encourage and facilitate my interest in historical preservation. That being said, a special thank-you goes to Al Cibelli, Mike Cook, Vivian Dellera, Elena Geonie, James Kilkenny, Elizabeth "Betty" Macchia, and all the retired Hudson River State Hospital staff whom I have known over the years. An immense appreciation is owed to Drew Scavello for his technical and photographic consultation; his backing in multiple historical projects has been critical. The biggest thank-you goes to my mother and father for always believing in me. Lastly, I could not ignore an early inspiration in documenting local history—John Leita and his wife, Laura Cummings; thank you for your work and friendship over the years.

Unless otherwise noted, all images are courtesy of the Hudson River State Hospital Nurses Alumni Association.

—Joseph Galante

Introduction

Mental illness was just gaining serious traction in the medical community as a disorder, juxtaposed to theories attributing causality to spiritual afflictions in the early 19th century. This was an era of social reform for the treatment of the poorer classes in society, specifically the insane and paupers. In 1827, Rev. Lewis Dwight, leader of the Boston prison reform movement, incited public consciousness regarding conditions of cruelty in American almshouses and jails, leading to boisterous societal outcries. Inspired by Reverend Dwight and time spent volunteering at the women's ward of the Cambridge Jail in Massachusetts, Dorothea Lynn Dix spent the remainder of her life in advocacy of the "insane." Dix, a teacher by trade, lobbied quite successfully and is credited in the development and expansion of over 40 state institutions for the mentally ill in the United States. Steadily conjoining societal views concerning the commonwealth's duty in dignifying the care of the insane began to grow both professionally and privately. In 1830, the New York State legislature would hear one of the earliest formal petitions addressing the conditions for "the insane poor" in the eastern region by surgeon Dr. Samuel White of Hudson. White was unsuccessful in swaying the men of the legislature to construct an asylum before returning to his practice in Hudson. However, he did establish his own private facility to care for the insane, which remained open until the construction and completion of the Utica Asylum. Dr. White became a point person of critical value in consultation for designing the state asylum at Utica. In 1844, White became a charter member of the Association of Medical Superintendents of the American Institutions for the Insane, commonly referred to as the "Superintendents Association," the first specific professional medical organization in the United States. White's work in formally characterizing the indigence the insane experienced to lawmakers was a prelude to the construction of the nearby Hudson River State Hospital.

The 1830s in Upstate New York was a time of economic prosperity and industrial growth on a size and scale that the region would never again see. Caring for the insane could no longer be overlooked, as industrialization was concomitant to a booming population. This growth led to the 1836 legislative resolve to begin work to establish an asylum at Utica, at the time slated to be the state capital. Admitting its first patient on January 16, 1843, the New York State Lunatic Asylum at Utica, as it was known at the time, became the first state-owned and -operated facility to care for the insane. Although this publication is about the Hudson River State Hospital, it is fundamental to understand the role of its predecessors in establishing the necessity and philosophy for constructing the hospital. During this era, the word *asylum*—derived from the Greek words *asyon* (meaning "refuge") or *asylos* (meaning "safe from violence")—had a more positive connotation. The Latin *asylum* means "sanctuary." It is important to contextualize that at this time, societally, the insane were treated as public spectacles to gawk at or mock. The Utica Asylum was postulated as a solution to the needs of New York's mental health system. The imposing stone structure was designed by William Clarke in the Greek Revival style and built on the pavilion plan, with four expansive, proportionate three-story buildings arranged in a quadrangle. Dr. Amariah Brigham was appointed superintendent of the asylum. In his first year in office, he published the *American Journal of Insanity*, describing treatments used in the facility and resulting outcomes. The first psychiatric journal of its type in the English language, it continues today as one of the most revered professional mental health journals, the *American Journal of Psychiatry*. Brigham was a charter member of the Superintendents Association alongside White. The 1840s were sharply different economically than the previous decade, as the county spiraled into its first depression. As a result, only one of the four originally proposed Utica Asylum buildings was constructed. The Utica Asylum had a two-year length of stay threshold, with few treatment modalities and limited space; subsequently, the facility became overcrowded.

Dr. Sylvester D. Willard, the New York surgeon general, was appointed to investigate the conditions of the insane living in county jails and poorhouses. In 1865, Dr. Willard noted deplorable, inhumane, and unsanitary living conditions for a staggering number of the insane. His report outlined in detail the overcrowding, cruelty, and lack of treatment so many county poorhouses exhibited. These findings, in conjunction with the overcrowding at Utica, guide the state legislature to commission two facilities to care for the insane of New York State, one to the east and one to the west. The first of the two constructed was the Willard Asylum for the Chronic Insane, about 109 miles to the southwest of the Utica Asylum. The main building at Willard, Chapin Hall, named after first superintendent John Chapin, was constructed based on the Kirkbride Plan, as Hudson River would also be. Across the American landscape, almost 50 Kirkbride Plan state hospitals were completed between 1848 and 1902. Named after Thomas Story Kirkbride, a young Quaker physician and superintendent of the Pennsylvania Hospital for the Insane just outside of Philadelphia, this model of care emphasized a building of equally proportioned wings to separate the sexes along with a central administration building. Careful consideration was given to maximize light and airflow for patients while limiting noise, in sharp contrast to the conditions found in poorhouses. The chief treatment was moral therapy: patients were encouraged to spend time on the parklike hospital grounds, work, sew, and engage in art and music as they labored toward recovery in the facility, a treatment leading to an ultimate goal of restoration to society. By the time Willard was completed in 1869, construction was under way on the Hudson River Asylum.

The emergent population resultant from industrialization and immigration in New York City amplified the need in the east for an asylum. Gov. Reuben Fenton appointed five commissioners under Chapter 666 of the Law of 1866 to locate a site for the eastern facility "on or near the Hudson below Albany." Waterways were largely the means of transportation at the time, so the position close to the Hudson River would allow for easy transport of goods and people, as eastern New York housed more than half the state's population. Poughkeepsie was ultimately chosen due to the consensus of the commissioners that the site should be central to railway and water in a large and active community. Governor Fenton and the legislature approved the resolve by virtue of Chapter 5 of the Laws of 1867; two hundred and eight acres of land between Poughkeepsie and Hyde Park were tendered as a gift from the citizens of Poughkeepsie and Dutchess County to serve as the site for the asylum. Legislation authorized the City of Poughkeepsie to borrow against its credit in the amount of $50,000 to purchase three-fifths of the Davis and Roosevelt family farms and allowed Dutchess County to borrow against its credit in the amount of $34,000 to purchase the remaining two-fifths of the farmland. The 200-plus-acre parcel of land, most of which was purchased from James Roosevelt, was a wooded expanse with rolling hills. Twenty-five acres on a plateau high above the Hudson River, which the *First Annual Report of the Hudson River State Hospital* calls "distinguished for its salubrity and commanding beauty," was chosen for the location of the first structures. Chapter 93 of the Laws of 1867 established and organized the hospital, which officially opened its doors that year as the Hudson River State Hospital for the Insane. Joseph M. Cleveland was appointed the first superintendent of the hospital, which had no facilities yet to receive patients. Remains from the Roosevelt family's Mount Hope, which burned in a fire that year, and farm buildings were all that stood. In 1869, renowned English architects Frederick Clarke Withers and Calvert Vaux were enlisted to design the hospital's main building based on the Kirkbride Plan. The grounds were a collaboration of landscape architects Frederick Law Olmsted and Andrew Jackson Downing, with influence from Vaux. Alongside these men, Dr. Cleveland worked to ensure an environment harmonizing treatment ideology with functionality and security. The main building was intended to house 300 patients of each sex in separate wings facing north and south, adjoined centrally by an administration building, with all the necessary kitchens, shops, and utility buildings in the rear of the main building to the east. It is imperative to consider how fully the state and medical community commended the Kirkbride philosophy of moral treatment by employing arguably the most influential men of their trades in developing this hospital. The main building, on the design of Vaux, Withers &

Co., was not completed until 1906. A colleague of this writer poignantly joked in 2000 during a presentation at Hudson River Psychiatric Center (at the time of the closing of the main building), "Could you imagine that fiscal constraints would influence the care of people?" Much like the proposed plan for the Utica Asylum, the main building at Hudson River State Hospital would never be brought entirely to fruition. This immense redbrick building, adorned with heavy stone trim and an ornate double-portico entrance of variegated brick, was built in the High Victorian Gothic style. From the inception of its design, Hudson River was criticized for "extravagance" by some in the government. State comptroller Nelson K. Hopkins remarked in 1871: "[For] refugees of the infirmed and distressed, the dependent classes in society, there seems to be no reason why any unnecessary expenditures should be allowed."

The board of managers sought to create, in correspondence with the philosophy of Dr. Kirkbride, a facility that furnished security for an asylum, refraining from generating a dull and oppressive environment for patients. The early years of the hospital were spent on construction and recruiting staff. On October 21, 1871, the Hudson River State Hospital admitted its first seven patients on order of transfer from the Utica Asylum. The facility dropped "for the Insane" from its name that year. Hope for recovery and reintegration into society was a standard operating procedure for patient care. Concurrently that October, three sections of the south wing male wards were completed, with the foundation for the fourth and final section being laid. The Hudson River State Hospital would have a catchment area consisting of 22 counties in eastern New York. By March 14, 1871, the hospital admitted 60 patients, a number that would steadily climb. Unlike previous facilities, Hudson River incorporated living quarters with single rooms in the main building to accommodate an average of 30 patients per ward. The board of managers for the hospital was not without obstacles in securing funds for constructing this dignified hospital for a less fortunate class. In retort to some accusatory claims of luxuriousness unwarranted to the insane, the Hudson River State Hospital Board of Managers stated in 1872:

> We are aware that by some persons the Hudson River Hospital is regarded as a much better-looking edifice then is needed for such a purpose. A building erected mainly for the poorer class cannot, they say, be too plain. To spend money in such a case, to only gratify the eye, is to waste it; in other words, it's sheer extravagance. For ourselves, we must acknowledge our inability to so view the matter, and our full persuasion that such opinions are not in accord with prevailing sentiment. We hold that no edifice of a public nature, and especially if conspicuously placed, of large dimensions and of a permanent character, should be put up in disregard to the aesthetic element.

The architecture of the building was intended to conjure an ambience of being cared for and valued in a hospital for treatment, not for confinement. The managers were able to accomplish construction of a hospital building reflective of the Kirkbride ideology while navigating the difficulties of being funded by a public budgetary department. Among the individuals appointed to the board of managers in 1873 was James Roosevelt, Esq., the father of Pres. Franklin Delano Roosevelt. The managerial board comprised local dignitaries who inspected the hospital for fulfillment in providing adequate treatment and living conditions. By 1883, Hudson River had a patient population of 308, comprising 165 males and 143 females. The hospital continued to grow in population as construction progressed. By 1890, the facility housed 900 acutely mentally ill patients. The year 1890 marked a landmark in mental health advancement. The State Care Act was signed into law, making New York State responsible for the boarding and treatment of the mentally ill, usurping the preceding system of individual county responsibility.

Chlorpromazine, marketed under the brand name Thorazine, introduced the first line of neuroleptic drugs to the world. The advent of this and other phenothiazine-based drugs caused many to believe mental illness could be managed effectively—so effectively, in fact, that it was assumed antipsychotics would act as insulin does to a diabetic. Sadly, the course of human history to follow would disprove this ideology. In 1955, Hudson River State Hospital was at a population of almost 6,000 patients. For a variety of reasons both good and bad, President Kennedy signed into law the Community Mental Health Act in 1963, creating the policy of deinstitutionalization nationwide. In modern times, deinstitutionalization is thought of as the policy of shuttering state mental hospitals. In actuality, that was not the intended goal of the bill. The goal was to provide more resources for treatment in the community, and as a by-product of available resources with improving treatment, the need for inpatient state hospitals would decline. Within the first few years of psychiatric medication being introduced, it was clear that it ameliorated the symptoms of mental illness for many individuals in life-changing ways. Many others, however, remained refractory to this treatment. Hudson River State Hospital was renamed Hudson River Psychiatric Center in the 1970s. The population of the hospital began to steadily decline and by 1984 was around 900. On January 25, 2012, Hudson River Psychiatric Center was officially shuttered after 145 years of dedicated operation. The facility was merged into Rockland Psychiatric Center, 65 miles to the south and just above New York City, where the remaining patients were subsequently transferred.

The face of mental health is forever changing. There is an inherent quality of any hospital or government system, and that is human design. To ignore the misfortunes or misdirections in the historical course of behavioral health would be irresponsible, but it is intellectually dishonest to perpetuate a widespread impression of a system constantly latent with malicious accounts of harm and neglect. It is the hope of this writer to impress upon the reader through the following images, taken mostly in situ over the course of the facility's life, the culture of care, dignity, and compassion. It is important to consider this when reflecting on the history of public behavioral health care after social reform in the 19th century; there is by and large no historical evidence that the bulk of caregivers or institutions were malfeasant or inflicted maltreatment on their charges. Over the course of its life, Hudson River Psychiatric Center was a model of progressive care around the country in pioneering improvements for the lives of psychiatric patients. Following a tradition of excellence in serving the mentally ill, Hudson River, although no longer officially the Hudson River Psychiatric Center, still provides quality outpatient care in several community living homes where individuals with mental illness continue to acclimate and adjust into broader society.

One
Establishment, Construction, and Growth

Beginning as a 208-acre parcel of land, the Hudson River State Hospital grew to encompass 752 acres acquired piecemeal. Opening initially as an independent building complex, the hospital constructed over five dozen separate buildings. Dr. Cleveland remained superintendent from organization in 1867 through 1893. His tenure witnessed the first shovel break the earth to bring forth the pencil-and-paper rendering of the institution. Due to failing health, in 1893, Dr. Cleveland tendered his resignation to the managers of the hospital, and he was succeeded by Charles Winfield Pilgrim, MD, a physician who worked at the Willard Asylum. Dr. Pilgrim advanced to assume the position of commissioner for the New York State Commission in Lunacy in 1917. Tremendous stories of the two superintendents knowing a remarkable number of patients on a personal level were commonplace. In 1929, in honor of Charles W. Pilgrim's service to New York State, Pilgrim State Hospital on Long Island, the world's largest state institution to date, was named to commemorate his amiability and dedication.

Initially, all services for patients were in the main building at Hudson River State Hospital. In 1889, construction on the first group of wards outside the main building was under way, and Central Group and Edgewood building opened to provide additional services. The philosophy was to create cottage groupings centered around small, individual farms. The produce would be sold in New York City markets to assist in financing the hospital. Additional cottages were furnished for patient living quarters requiring minimal security in 1891. Around the turn of the century, a power plant, butcher shop, piggery, barns, various trade shops, water and sewage treatment plants, icehouse, broom shop, shoe shop, and mattress shop, to name a few, were operational.

By 1994, Harlem Valley and Middletown Psychiatric Centers were consolidated in Hudson River. The final chapter in the life of the historic old main building came in 2001, as the facility closed its "lower campus." Director Carol Stevens was the final woman in a long series of individuals to govern the hospital. The light switches were turned off at Hudson River Psychiatric Center for the final time on January 25, 2012.

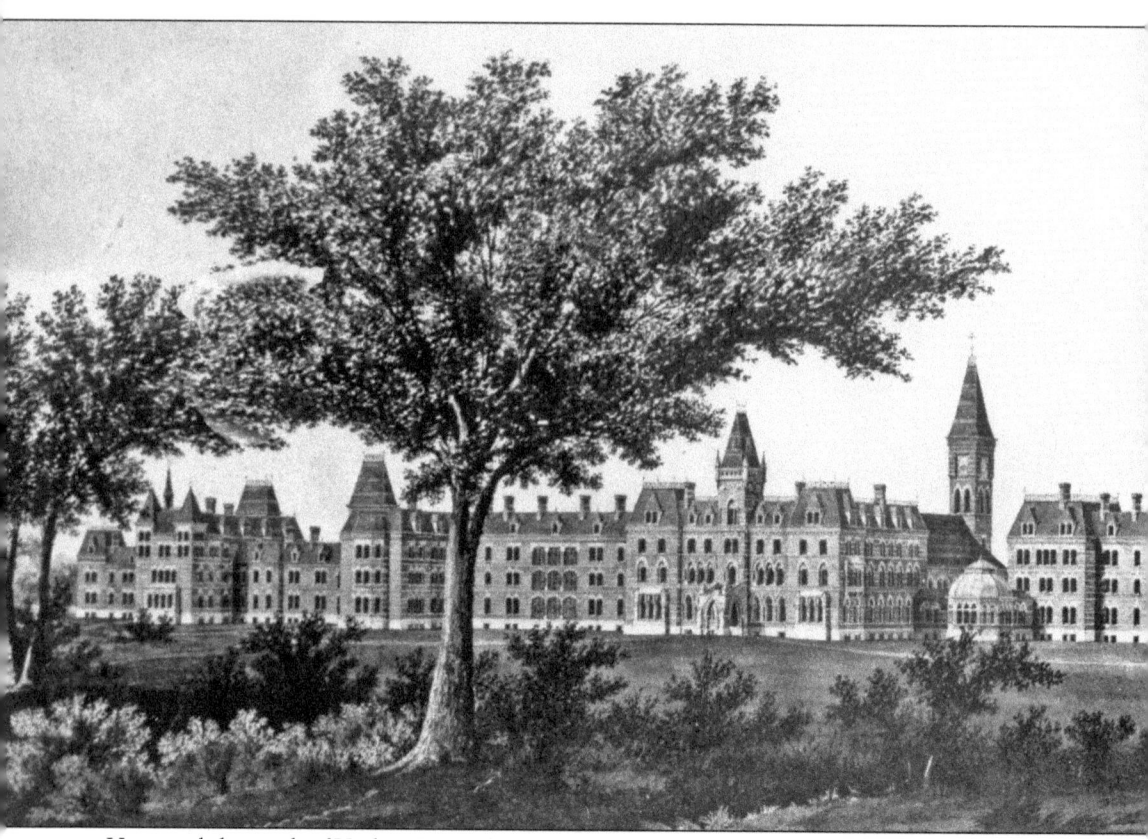

Here is a lithograph of Hudson River shortly after opening in 1874. At the time this was published, another Kirkbride Plan state hospital was under way at Buffalo as well as one at Middletown to homeopathically treat patients. The picturesque work of Olmsted's parklike lawn in the foreground is eye-catching. Before drafting his most prominent creation, Central Park in New York City, Olmsted practiced at several state institutions around the country in a similar style. Rolling hills

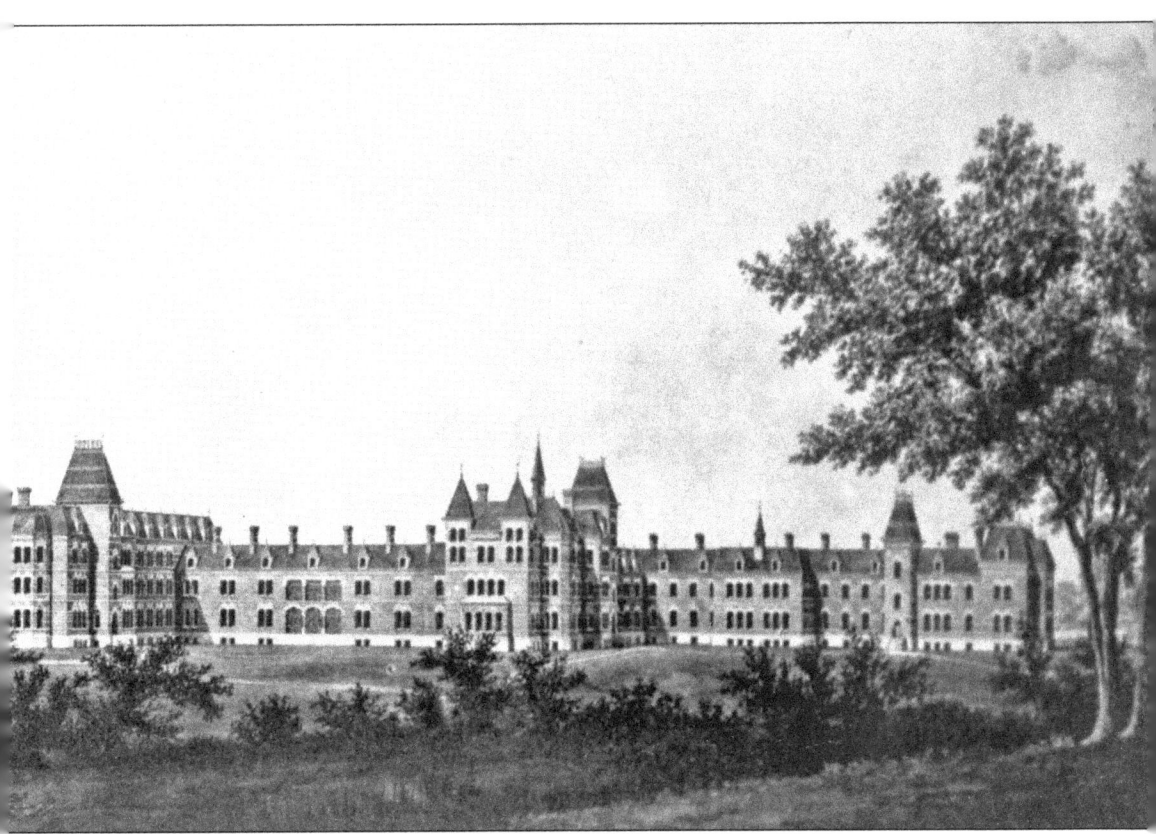

with winding walkways similar to those of Central Park were part of Olmsted's vision for Hudson River's grounds. The ornate stonework and natural proportions of the main building reflect the Victorian Gothic beauty one would find on Broadway in New York City. This lithograph appears in the February 1874 issue of *Harper's Weekly*, a highly viewed source of socially important news at the time.

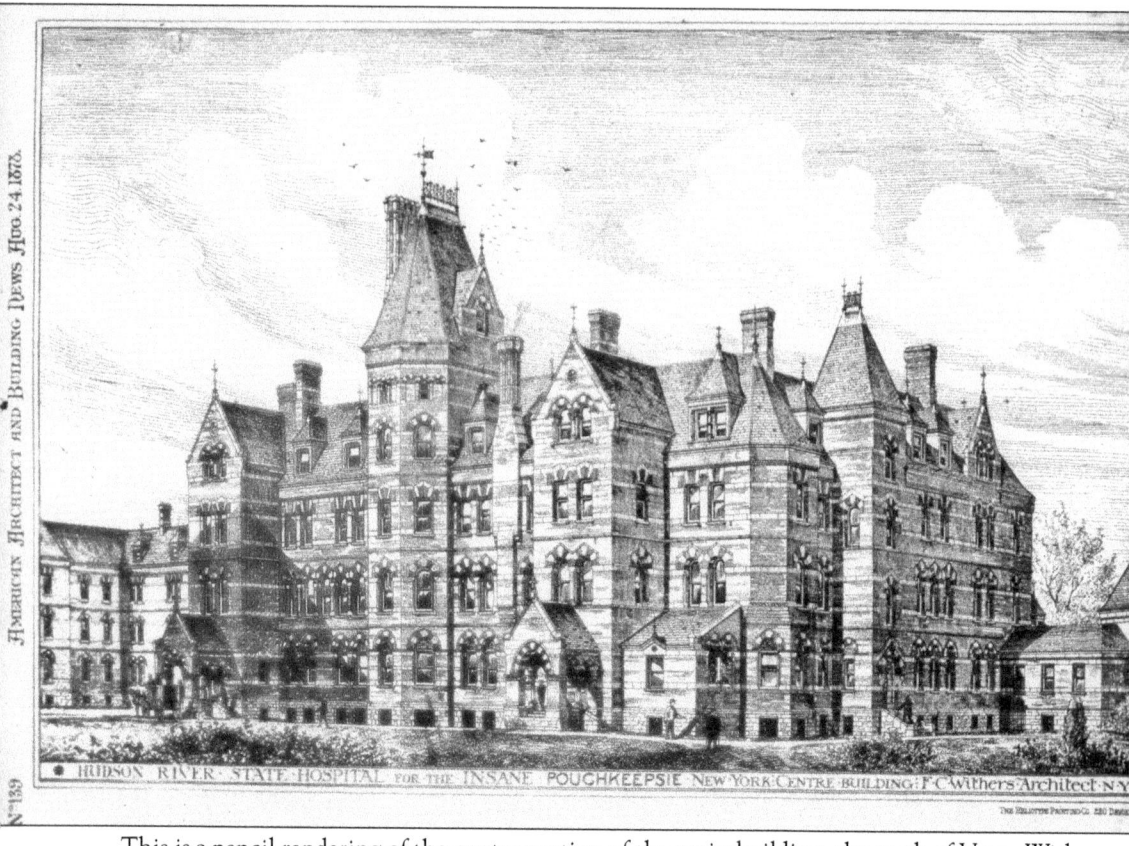

This is a pencil rendering of the center portion of the main building, the work of Vaux, Withers & Co. employing the ideals of the Kirkbride Plan. The managers remarked in 1871: "Generally it has been thought of as a matter of considerable importance to put up a cheerful, liberal first impression in connection with that main entrance of the building. . . . It gives diversity and brightness to the whole exterior and relieves the eye of which would be weary of a vast momentous red expansion." This was critical for the founders, including Dr. Cleveland, who were aware of the role of environment in treating patients. Security needed to be furnished in this building because of its purpose, but this was done in a way that the features providing that condition were not salient. The administration building being the first sight of patients and visitors made it a prominent focal point, overtly projecting the appearance of a curative facility, not an oppressive one.

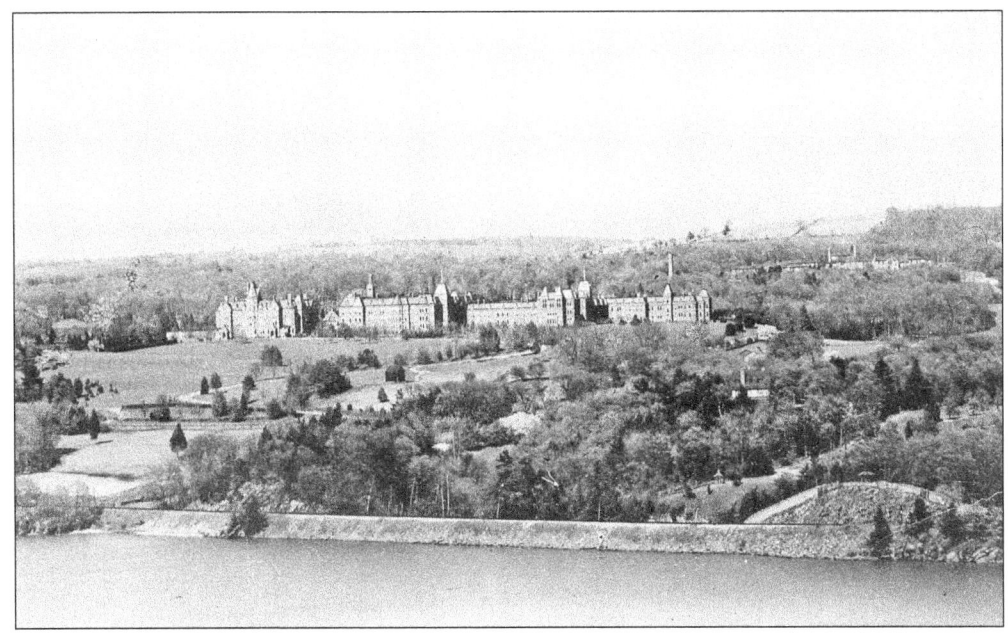

A view of the main building from across the Hudson River is shown in this mid-1890s image. Note that the north wing, later located left of the center building, was not yet constructed. With no trees mature enough to block a complete view of the structure, the size and grandeur of the design are quite salient. In the background, the Central Group can be seen.

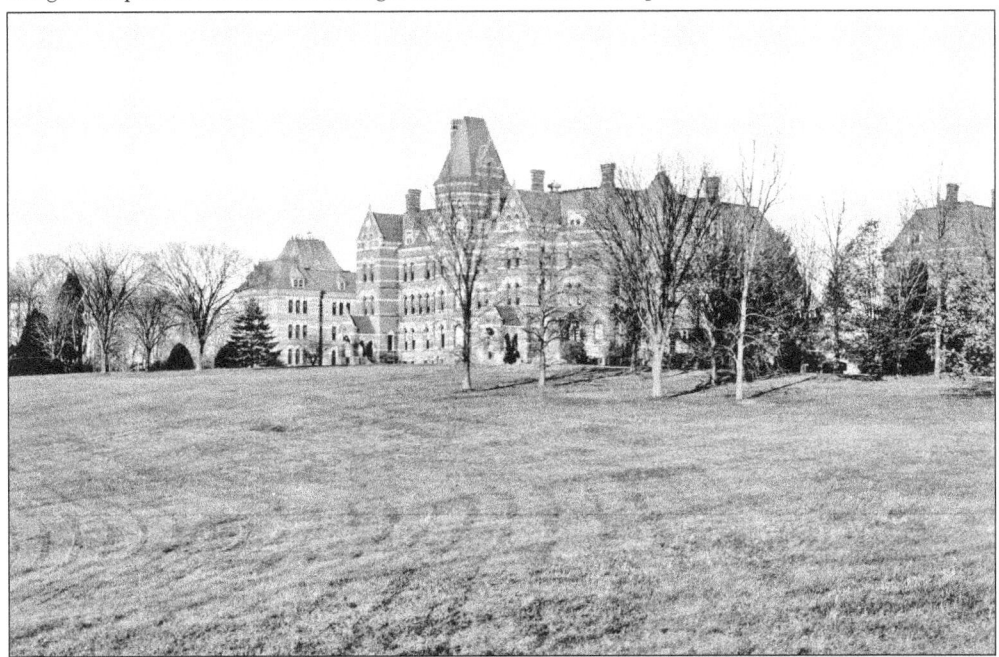

Juxtapose this image with the previous photograph of the main building. This mid-1910s image taken from the lawn in front gives a clear view of the center administration building. Note the north wing's mansard roof jutting out to the far left; this wing of the building had not been constructed yet when the previous image was taken. The neatly manicured lawn in the foreground was a typical sight at Hudson River.

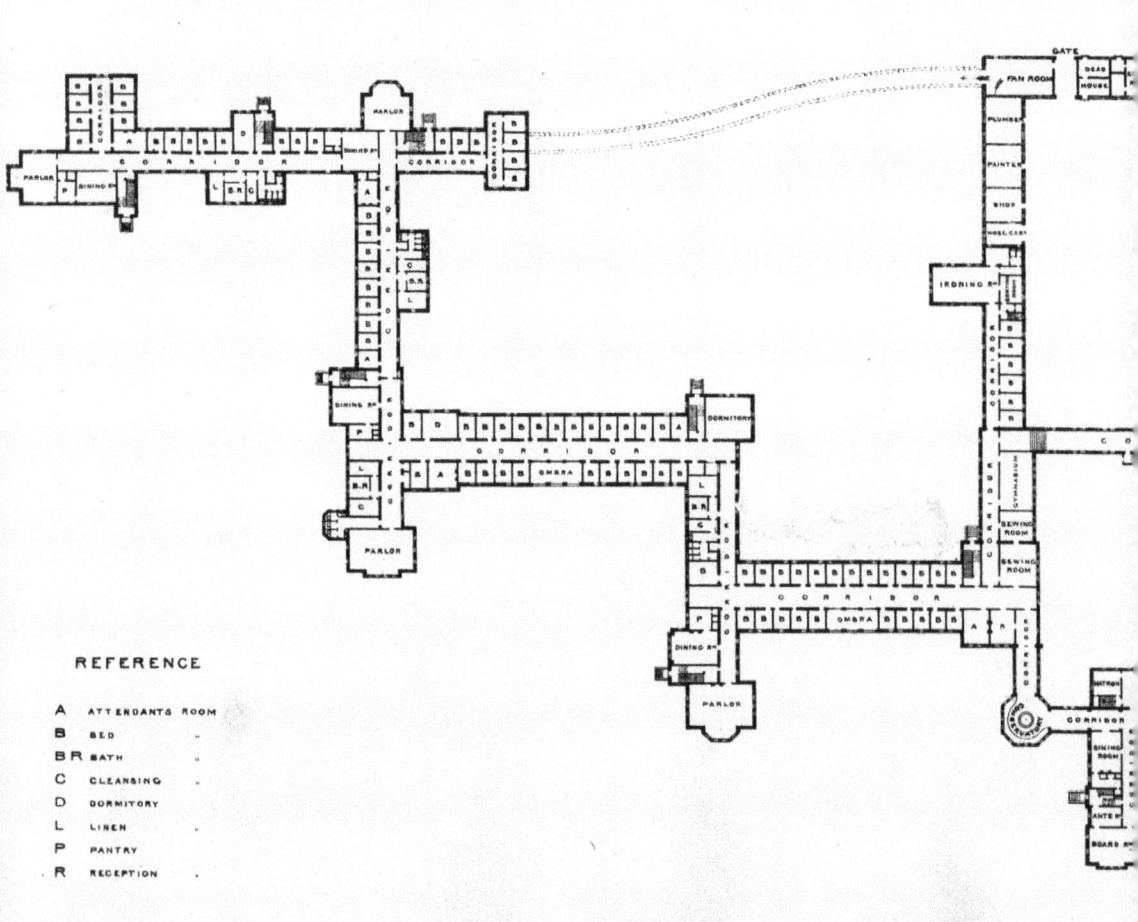

This is the original 1867 Vaux, Withers & Co. floor plan for the main building. The intended design called for two wings of equal dimensions to house separate sexes. Fiscal constraints over the course of erecting this building, along with later shifting ideologies of hospital construction, made Hudson River State Hospital possibly the only Kirkbride Plan hospital in the United States

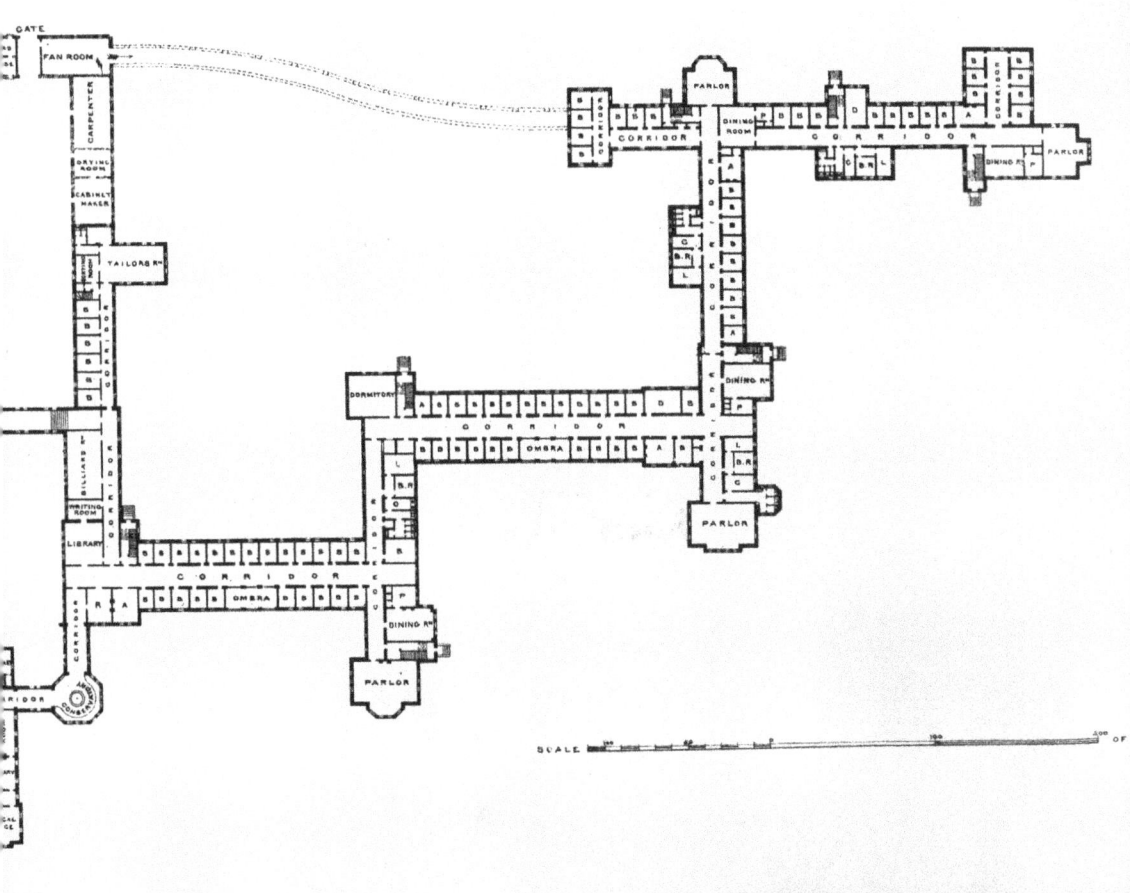

not initially completed in parallel proportions. The main structure consisted of the central administration building and south wing until 1898, when the north wing was added. By 1906, construction was officially completed on the main building complex, which never received the last two ward blocks on the north wing.

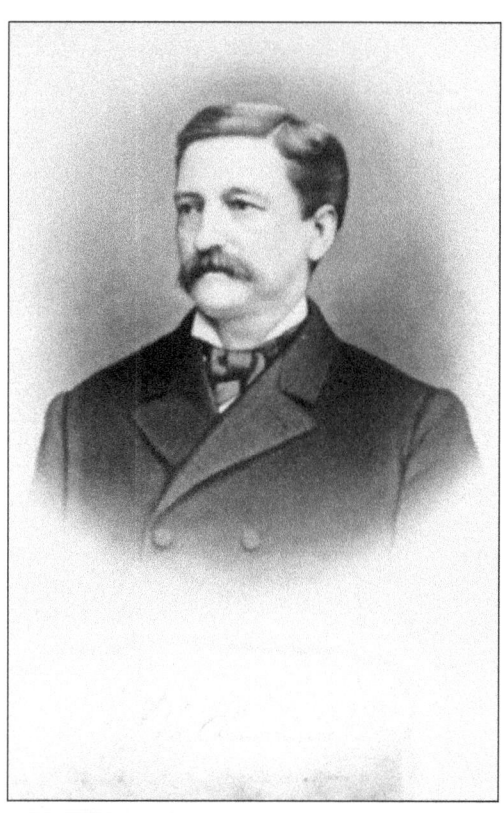

Dr. Joseph M. Cleveland was appointed the first superintendent of Hudson River State Hospital in 1867. He had specialized in the nuances of public mental health care at the Utica Asylum. Schooled in the principles of humane and moral treatment Dr. Amariah Brigham established at Utica, Dr. Cleveland continued a tradition of high standards of care and living for all patients under his charge at Hudson River.

This is a typical ward in the north wing of the main building around 1900. This wing was still exclusively utilized for female patients. Common areas were unlocked during the day, allowing patients to move freely about the ward. They could socialize in the day hall, go to program areas, or find a spot to perhaps knit on one of these hallway benches. Wards for more disturbed patients had far fewer items publicly available and were housed in the Central Group by 1891.

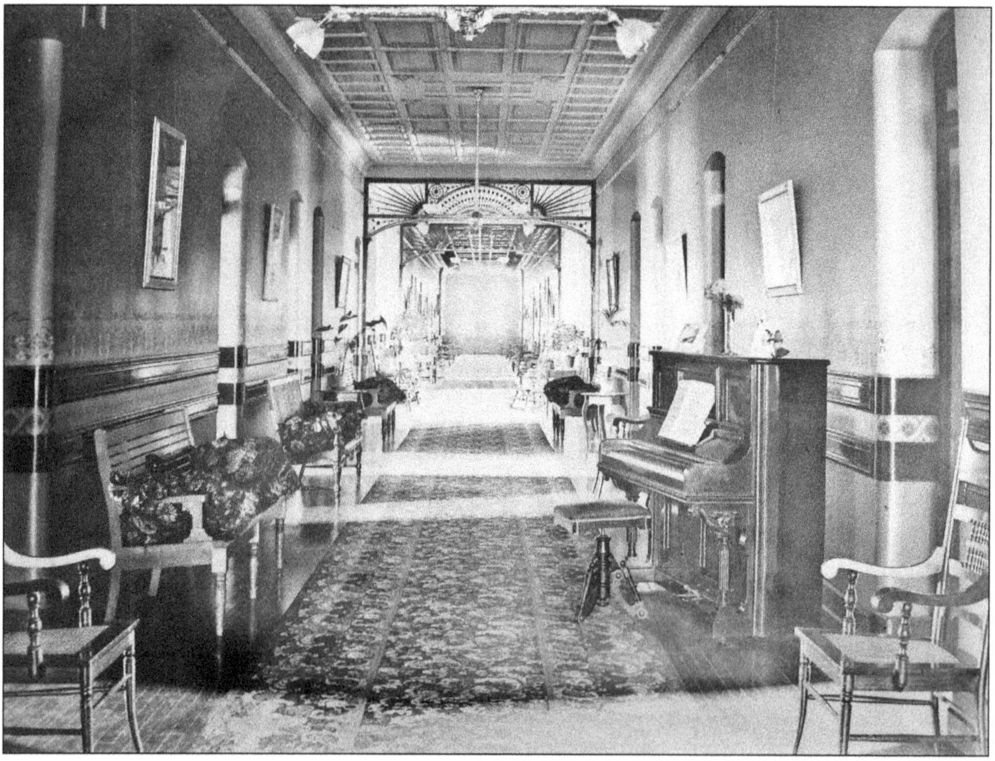

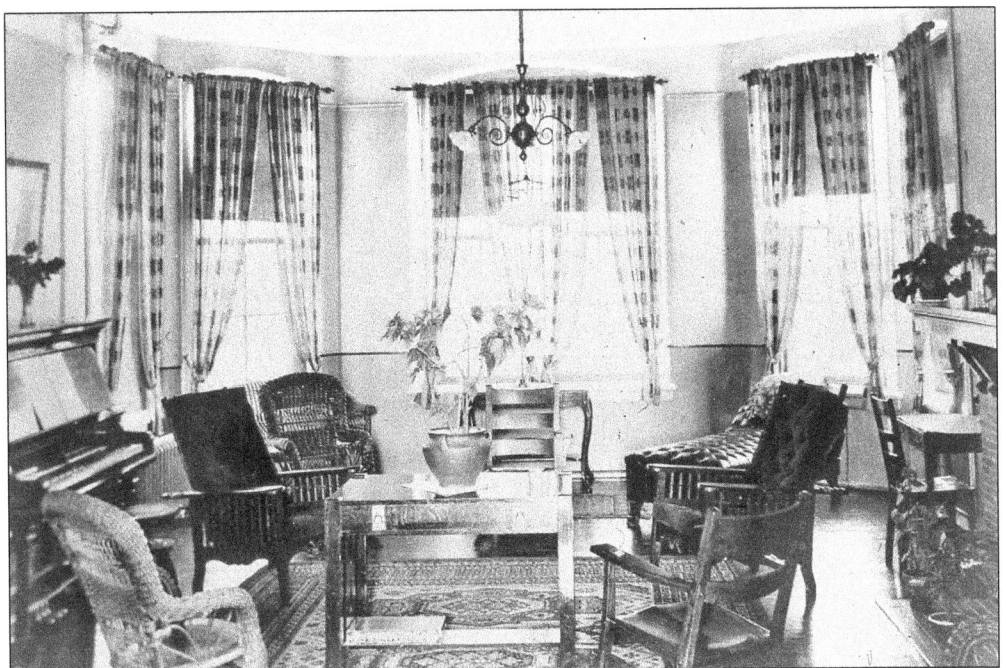

Outside of the larger day halls on some of the wards in the main building were smaller alcoves like this one in the south wing. Here, a smaller group of individuals could gather and socialize or enjoy the music of a piano without interrupting other activities in the larger day hall.

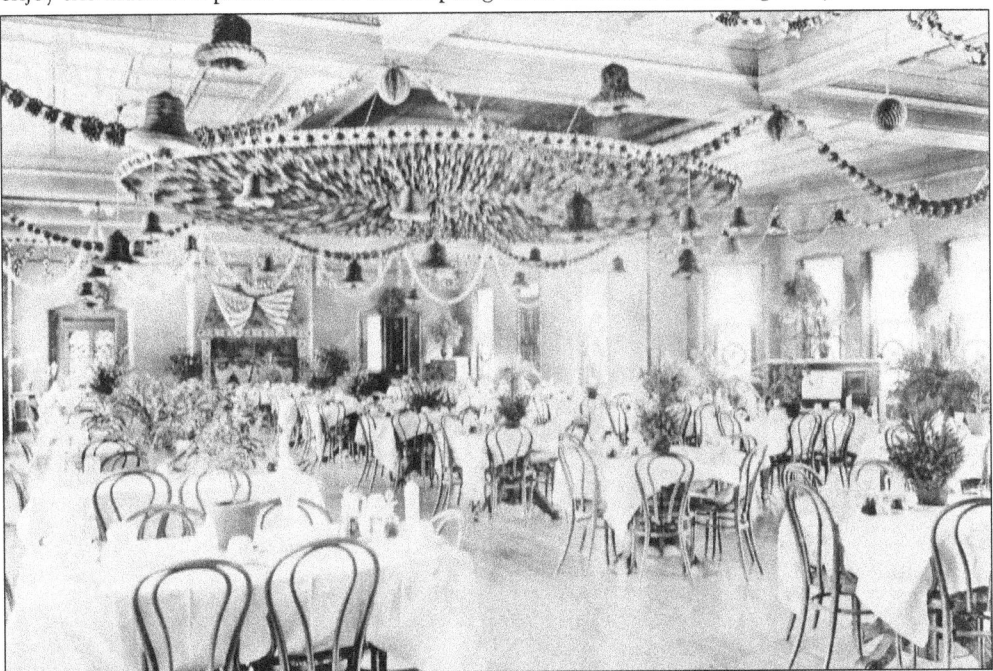

This photograph was taken at the close of the 19th century just prior to a Christmas celebration in the attendants' dining hall in the north wing. Staff and patients often celebrated holiday festivities together. In these times, staff lived in the same building as patients, who were down a separate ward hallway.

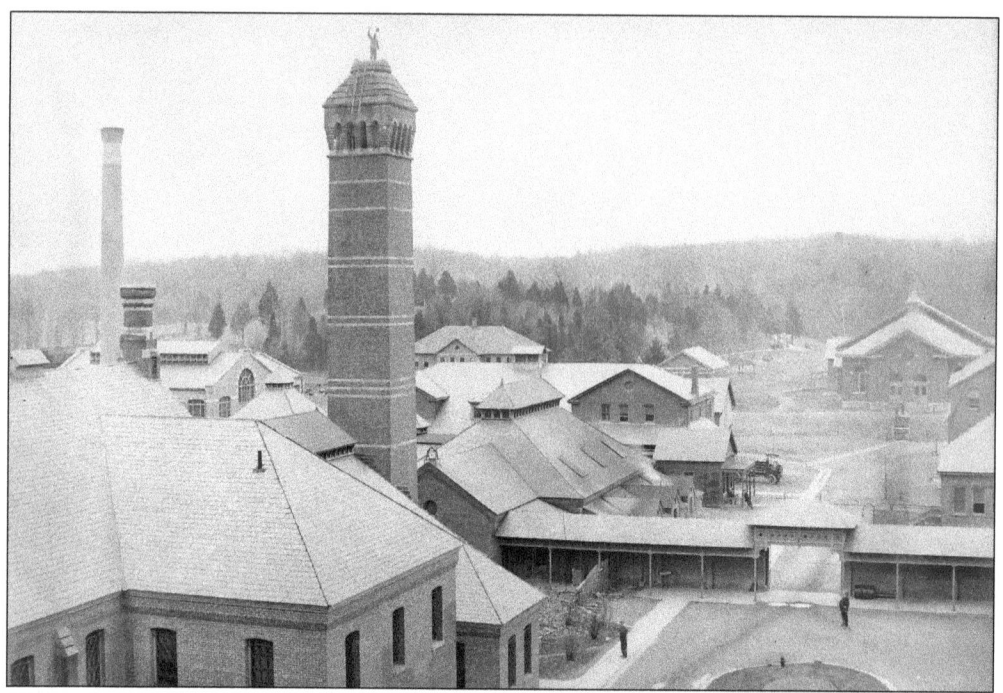

This early 1900s photograph was taken from the center building of the main building complex. In view are all the shops, the laundry, the boiler, and the power plant that maintained the hospital. Atop a chimney, a maintenance man can be seen inspecting the condition of the chimney as his colleagues watch from the ground.

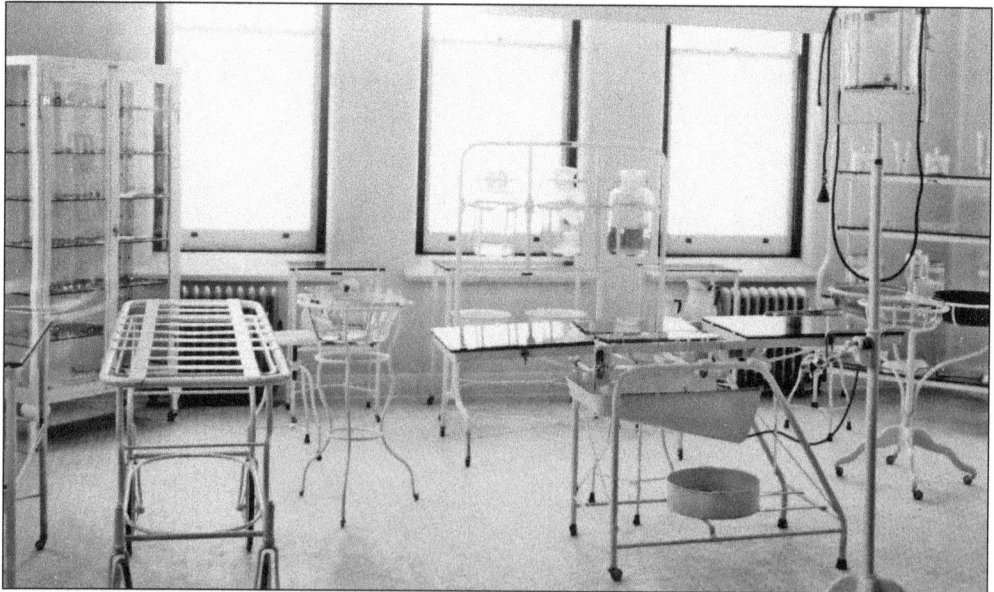

Before the construction of an independent infirmary in the Brookside building, medical and surgical services were located on a ward in south wing. This 1912 photograph shows the "modern" operating room in the main building for both staff and patients requiring surgical intervention. Because electricity was in its infancy, note the large windows in the background for light; these would not be found in an operating room today.

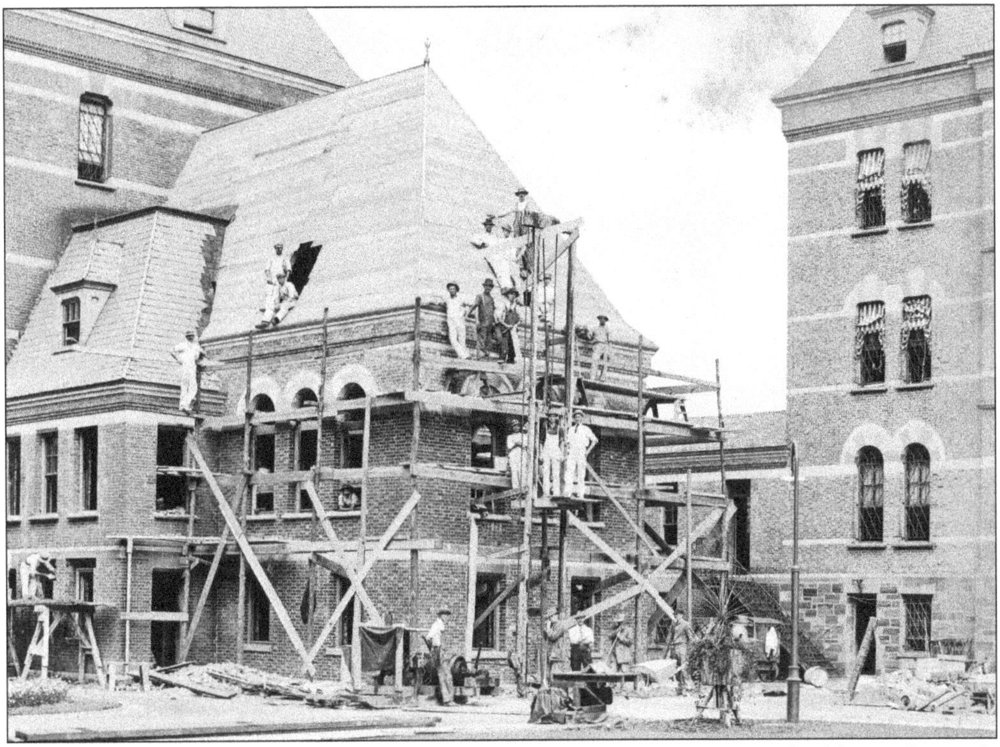

Over the years, many renovations and additions were made to the main building. This early addition in the 1910s took place on the rear of the center of the main building. Careful attention was paid to match the existing materials and style of the building. In later years, this segment of the building was utilized as the credit union.

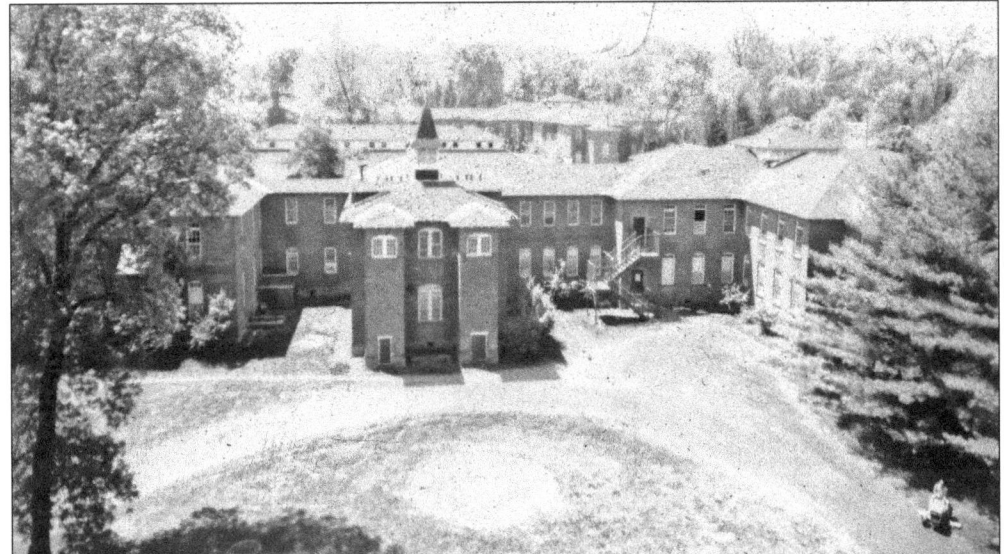

The Central Group was erected in 1889 and served as the first cluster of buildings outside the main building for patient care. This complex was to the southeast of the main buildings in a seclusive area of the hospital property. It was built to accommodate the growing number of patients at Hudson River and alleviate overcrowding in the main building.

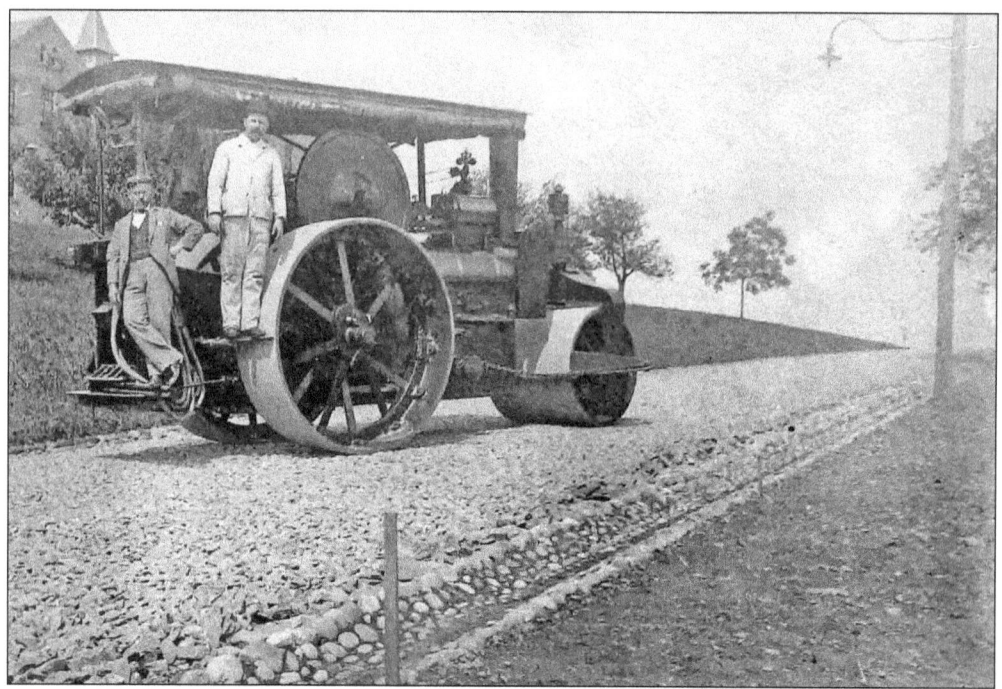

Hudson River State Hospital was a self-contained and autonomous facility for the majority of its operating life. This 1910s photograph shows farmers aiding in the construction of roads with a steam-powered machine on the grounds of the hospital. Stone for this construction was quarried on-site and transported via horse and carriage.

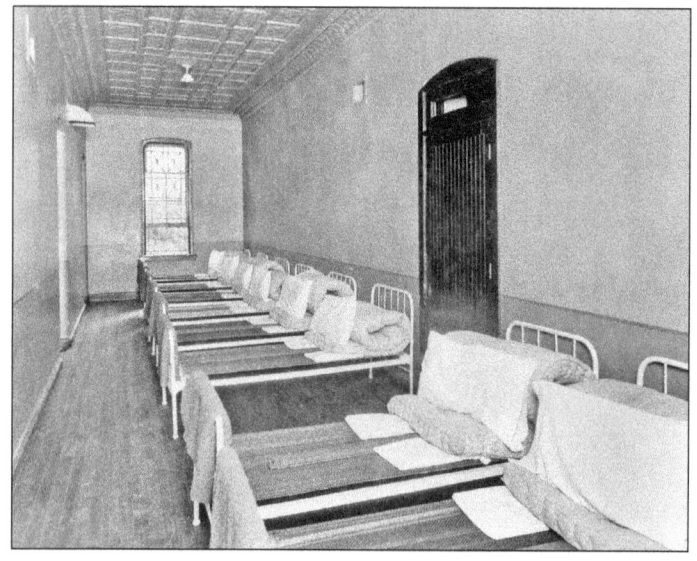

This image was taken from a ward filled beyond capacity in the south wing of main building in the early part of the 20th century. This ward housed only men at the time. Hospital administration worked to ensure that with a growing population, the treatment and housing services grew as well. Take note of the spotless quartersawn pine floors and decorative painting around the chair rail molding in this dormitory hallway.

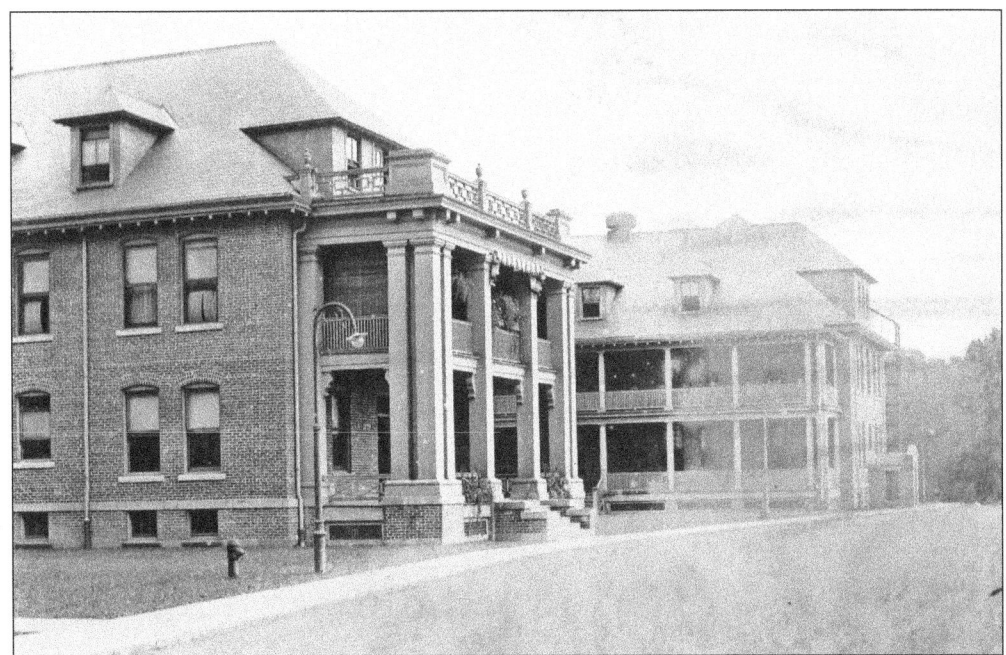

The Inwood building was completed in 1906 to house and treat the chronic cases of the hospital. These were patients who had been psychotic for some time and whose prognosis towards a recovery was nil. Inwood was designed to house 440 individuals suffering from various mental afflictions.

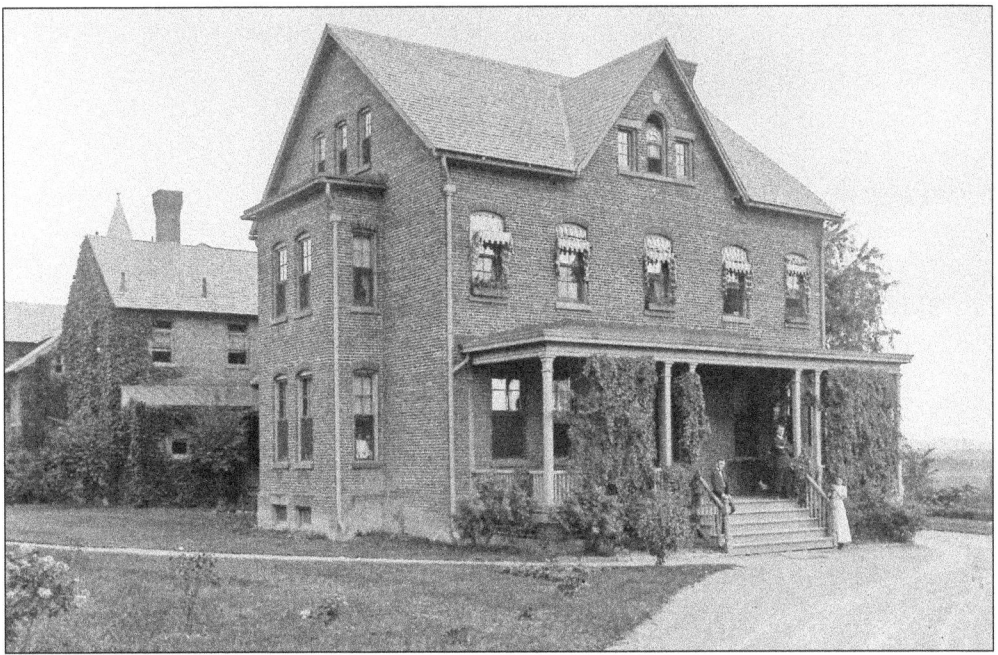

Not all patients lived on wards that were locked at all times. "Honors patients" or "patients with keys" were terms for patients who posed little to no worry of escape or injury. They found more private accommodations in the cottages like the one shown here, which had single-room living. Most of these patients came and went about as they pleased during day hours. The cottages were generally locked at night.

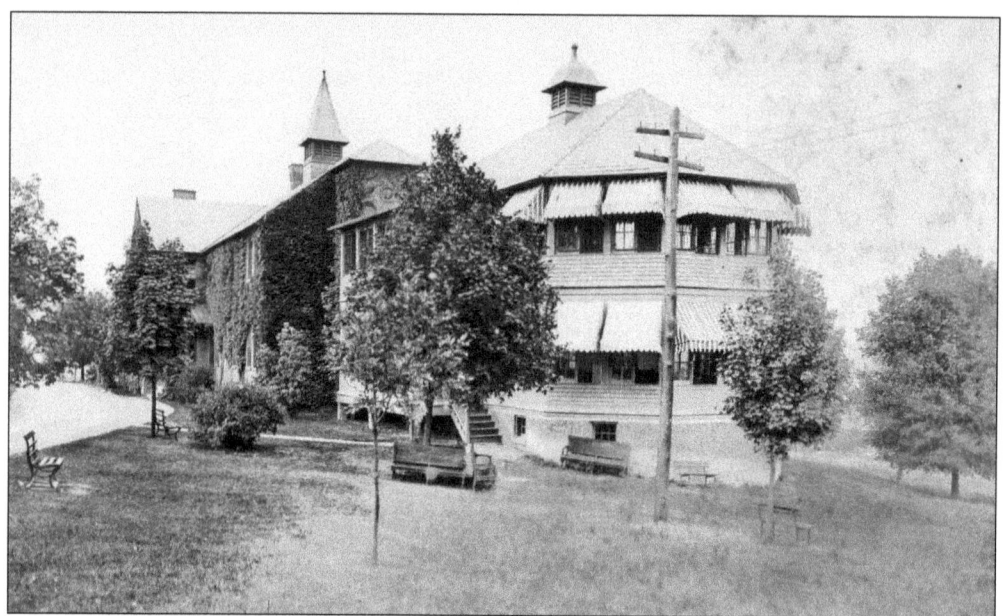

For the lower-security cottages, sunporches made mainly of glass were constructed, like the one shown here at Cottage 6 in the Central Group around 1918. Patients could enjoy sun and fresh air in the summer as well as cozy winterscapes thanks to steam heat. If close observation is made to the windows, it is clear that no security features preventing escape exist.

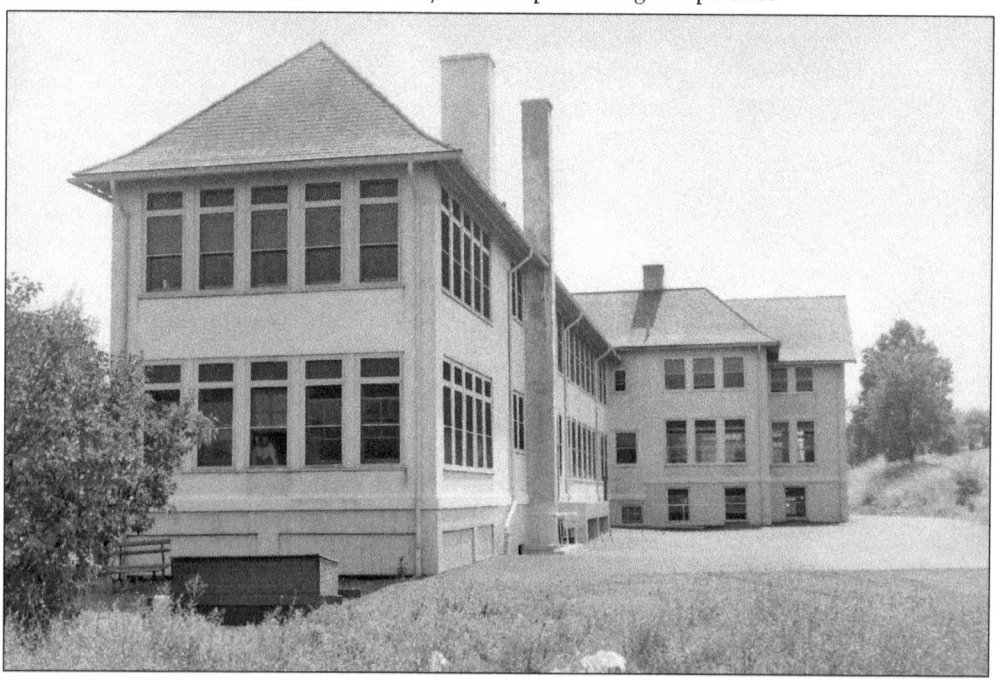

As tuberculosis became rampant in the earlier part of the 20th century, it was imperative to quarantine patients afflicted with the disease. A building with excellent ventilation and airflow was critical to reduce chances of passing the illness to those not infected. The Lakeview building was constructed to serve as a TB treatment ward in 1922. Prior to its construction, two cottages in the Central Group were used to segregate TB patients beginning in 1893.

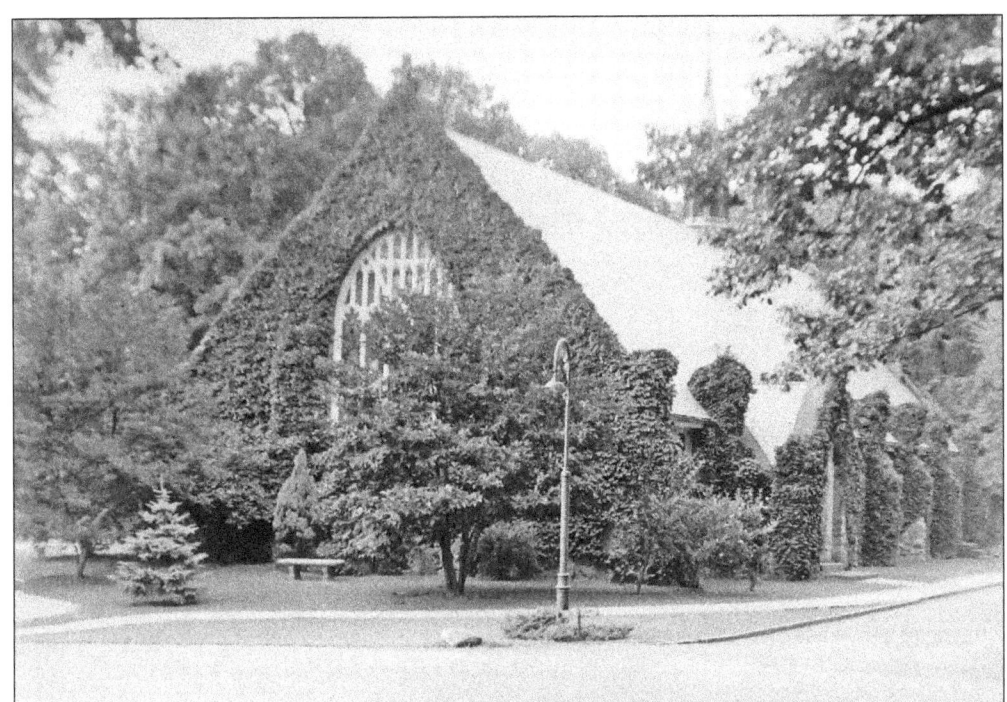

The first freestanding building for worship at Hudson River, Our Lady of the Rosary Catholic Church, was constructed in 1906. Still in operation as a private church today, this edifice was erected on donation from the Smith family of New York City, the makers of Smith Brothers' Cough Drops. The church was dedicated in memory of Sister Ann Smith, a daughter of the millionaire family who took the vow of poverty to become a nun. When she left to take her vows, Ann's father was furious and cut her off from the family fortune. In those days, entering a convent meant almost never returning home. At her father's passing, all were shocked to find out that Ann received an equal inheritance with her brothers. Her brothers felt a church to serve the mentally ill would be a noble remembrance.

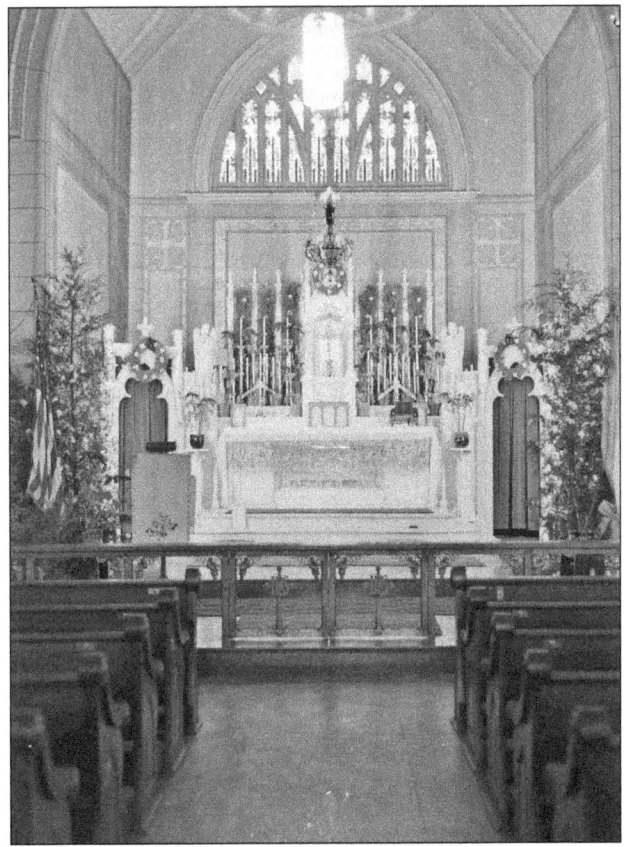

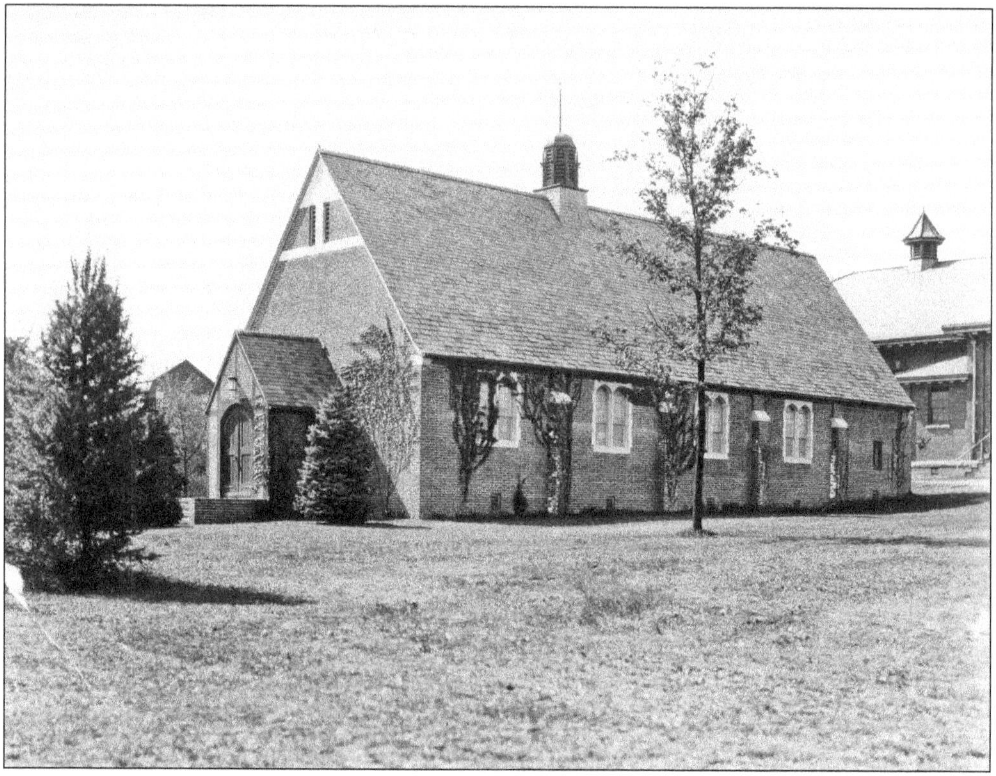

A second chapel, Avery, was constructed in 1926. This brick-and-mortar structure was named for Martha Avery, a dignitary on the hospital's board of managers. This was a freestanding building that patients could leave their wards to visit. Religious worship was held near and dear to many patients, especially those with no family to turn to in their times of need.

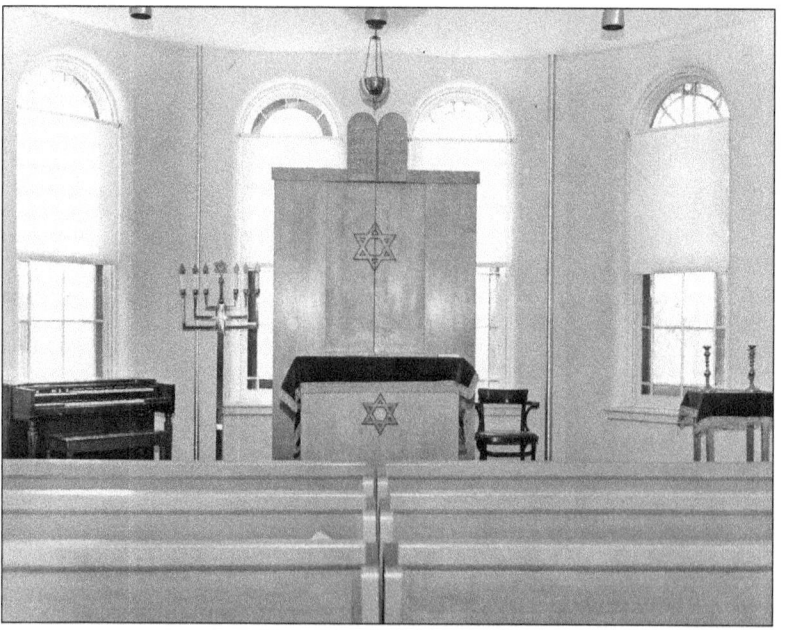

Jewish religious services were made available to staff and patients who practiced their faith at Hudson River. This synagogue was constructed in the south wing of the main building as room was made available on a repurposed ward located close to the center building. This photograph was taken around the 1960s.

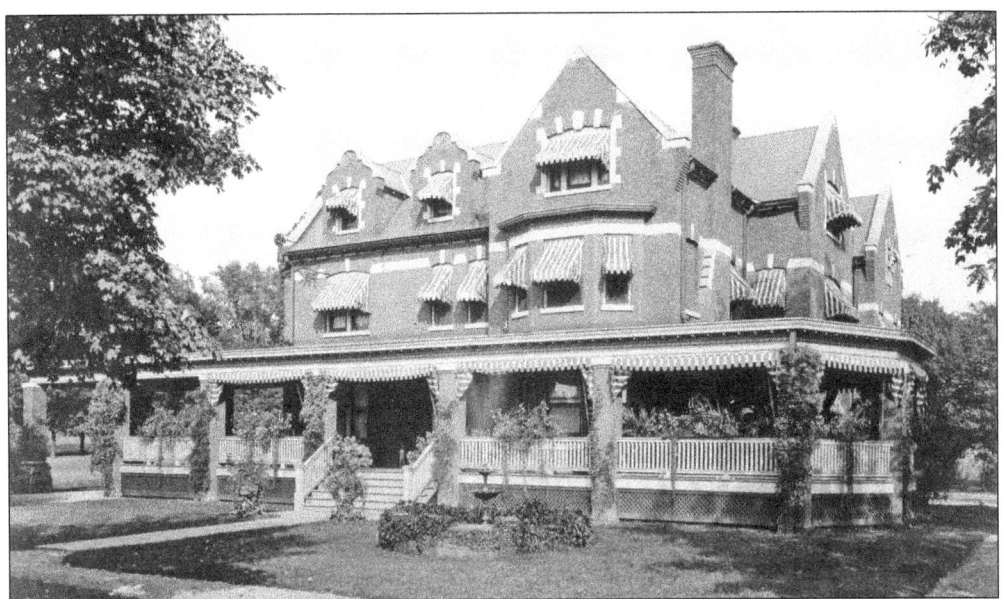

Being superintendent of the hospital was not without its perks. This is the superintendent's mansion, occupied in 1906. Quartering in this large private residence was part of the terms of employment for the position. Housekeeping, groundskeeping, and general maintenance were part of the package. Prior to this separate house, the superintendent had an apartment on the third floor of the administration portion of the main building.

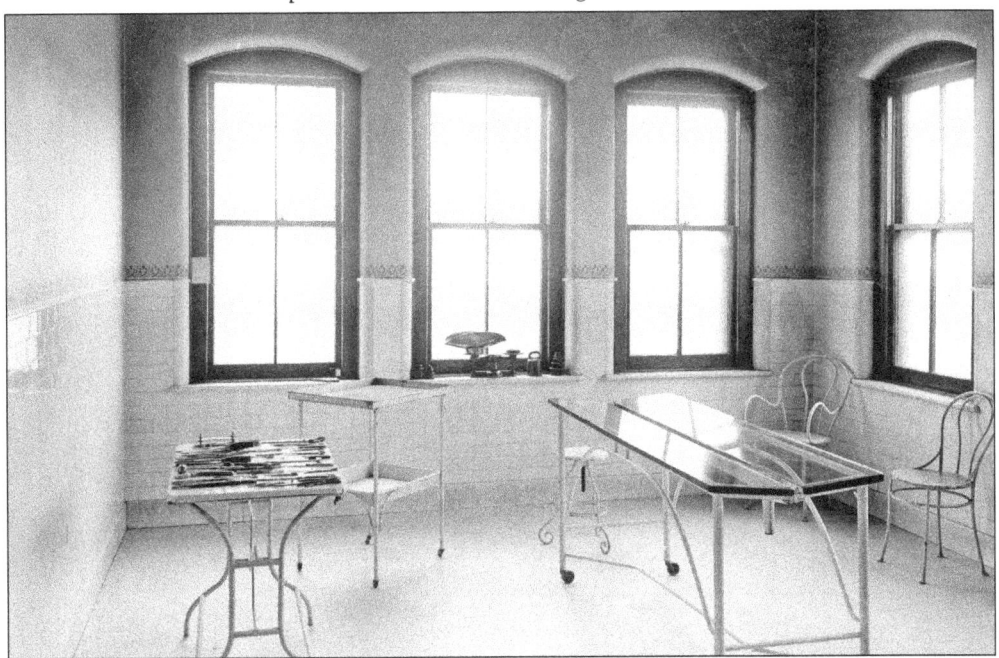

A small square-shaped building behind the main building served as the hospital's morgue and laboratory since 1896. From the earlier days of mental health to the present, cadaver study of the human brain has allowed for a learning curve in regard to the biology of mental disease. Such examination could not be done on a living person. This building was state of the art at the time it opened. This early image shows the autopsy suite, where postmortem examination took place.

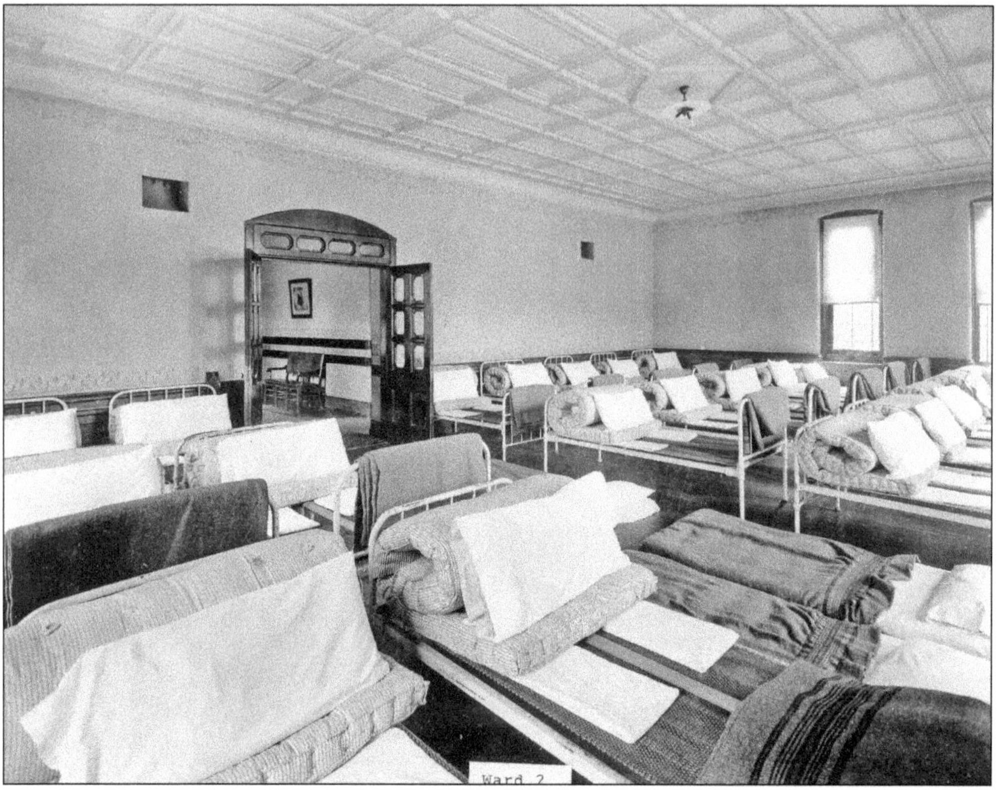

As the population increased at Hudson River, space for lodging individuals had to be fully utilized. Wards designed for comfortably housing 30 patients in the old main building grew to accommodate 50 or more. This 1905 photograph shows a crowded dormitory in the south wing of the main building.

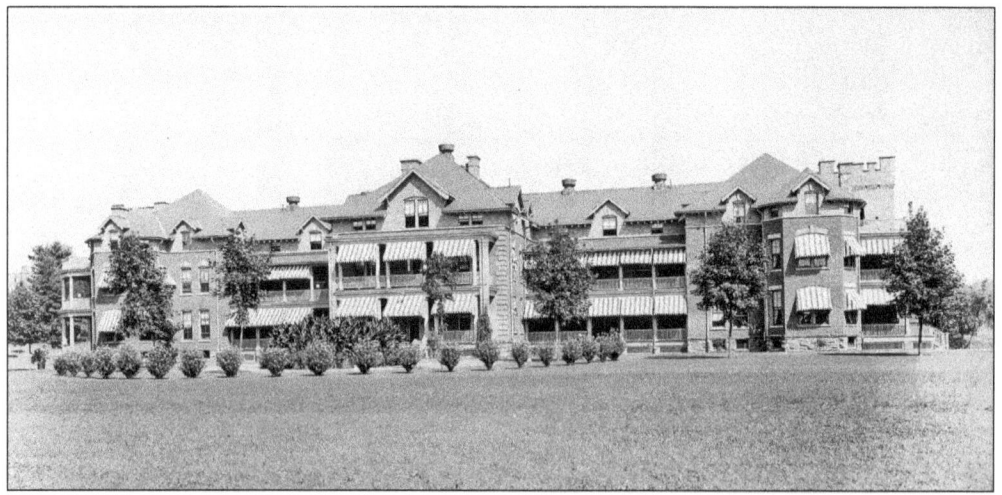

Pilgrim Hall was dedicated on May 1, 1917, in honor of Dr. Pilgrim, the second director of Hudson River. Pilgrim Hall served as the admitting building from its opening on December 22, 1908, through the early 1960s. Here, patients were diagnosed and placed in the appropriate building. In the foreground is one of the many gardens patients and staff would maintain on the grounds of the hospital as part of therapeutic recreation and activity.

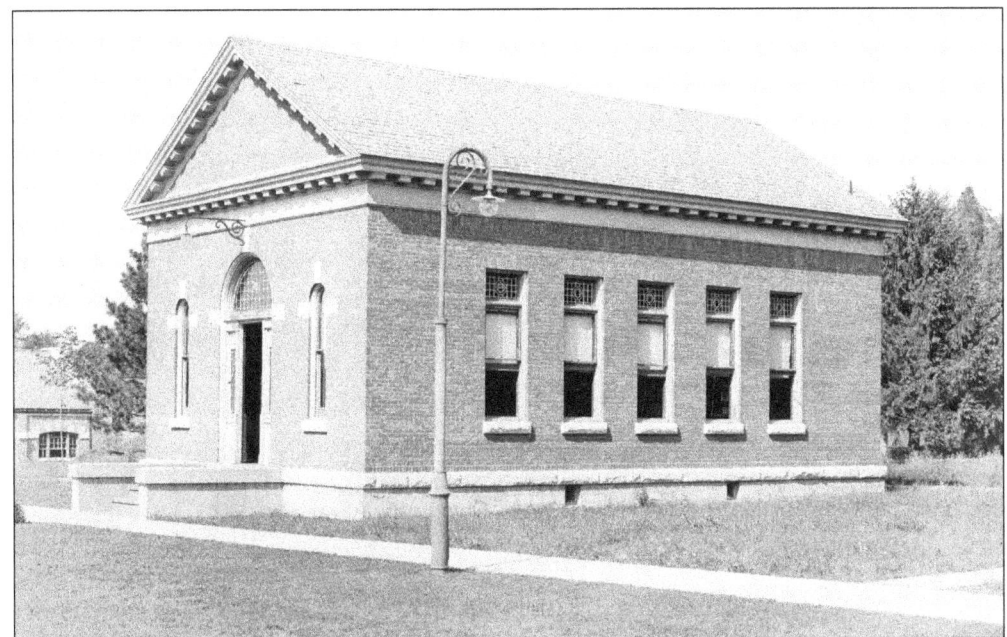

A freestanding patient library opened in 1910 for those with privileges to leave the wards. It was behind the main building, next to the theater building. For those who could not leave their wards, the librarian would take books on a cart and make trips around the buildings. This was a task often aided by a patient-worker.

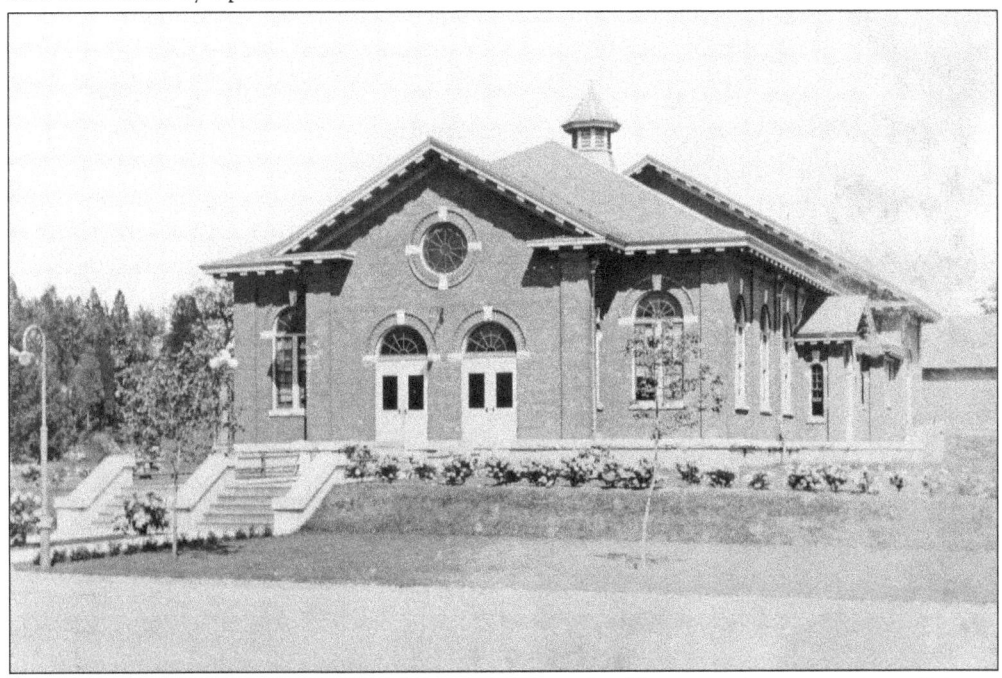

Recreation and activities were thought to be of considerable importance to patients living a fulfilling life. This amusement hall opened in 1905 for entertainment and physical activity. It contained a stage, movie theater, basketball court, and gym for cooperative movement, dances, and social events.

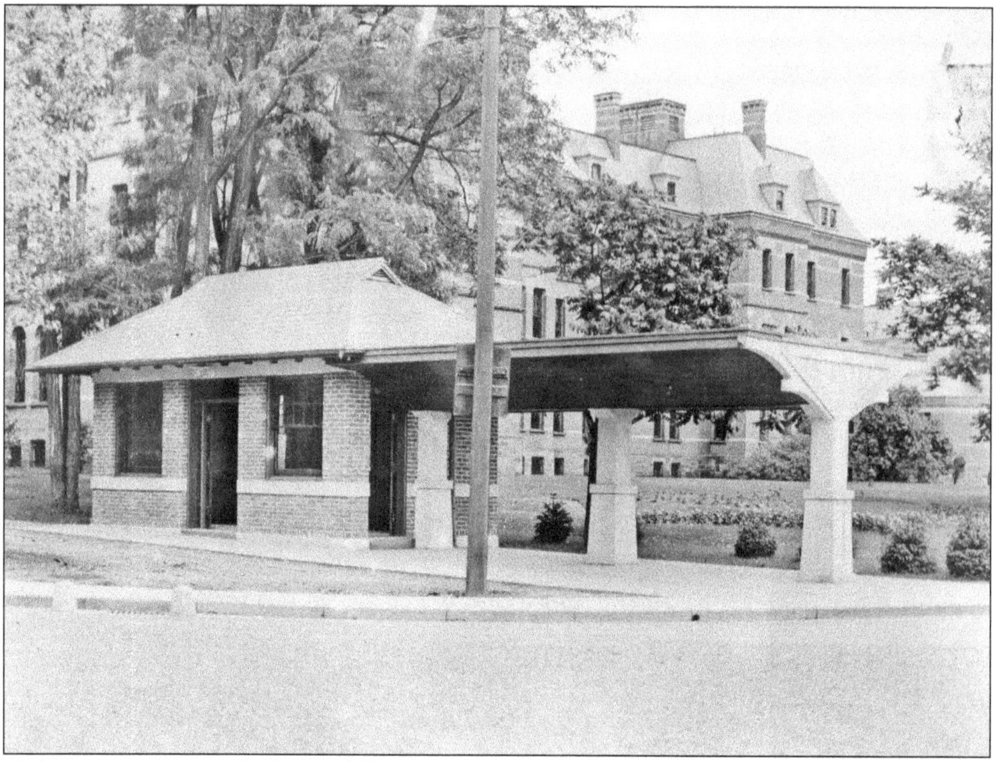

To bring visitors up to the hospital from the nearby rail line, a trolley with service to the hospital was made publicly available. Visiting days in the earlier times of the hospital were Wednesdays and Saturdays. The waiting station pictured here, originally utilized as a trolley stop, in later years became a snack canteen frequented by patients.

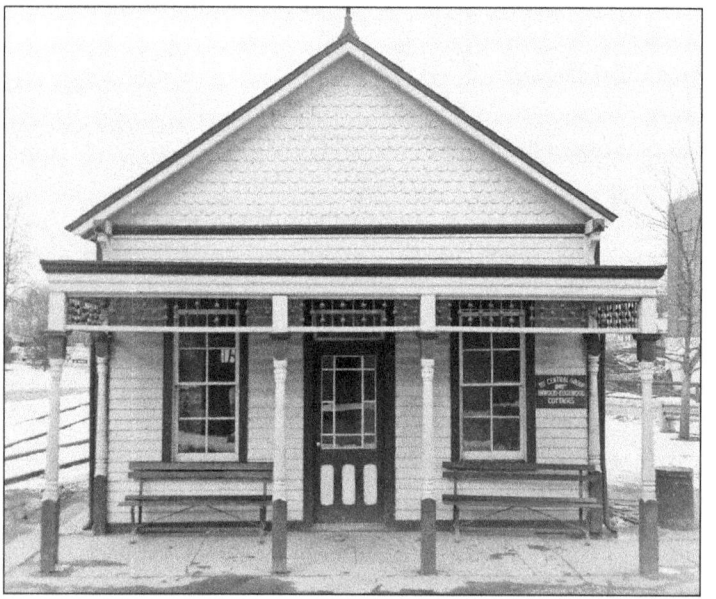

As the grounds grew over the years, it became a sizable walk between certain buildings. For those who were elderly or infirm, this was especially a challenge. Many patients had privileges to travel the grounds unescorted from one building to another for groups, work, or leisure. This bus stop allowed individuals who had a hard time with distance to retain their independence and/or provided plain convenience of travel.

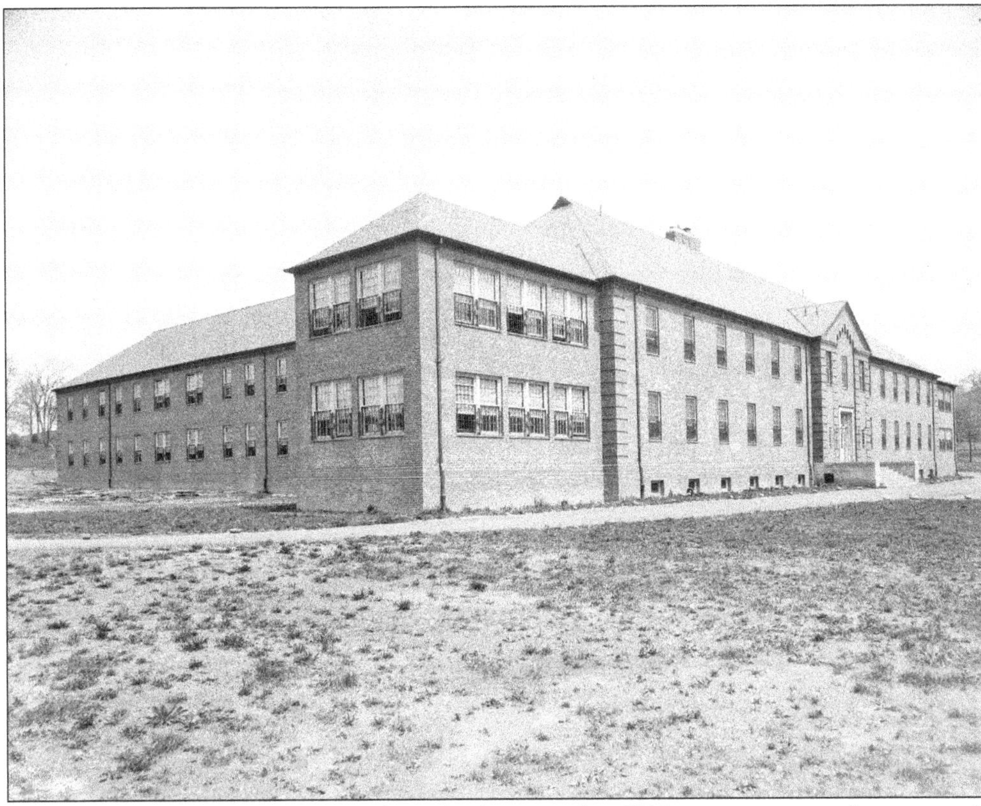

The infirmary building, later named Brookside, opened in 1930 to serve as a modern center for medical and surgical services. This was the first freestanding building constructed at Hudson River to act solely as an acute medical hospital. In the past, only individual wards for such a purpose existed in the main building and the Central Group.

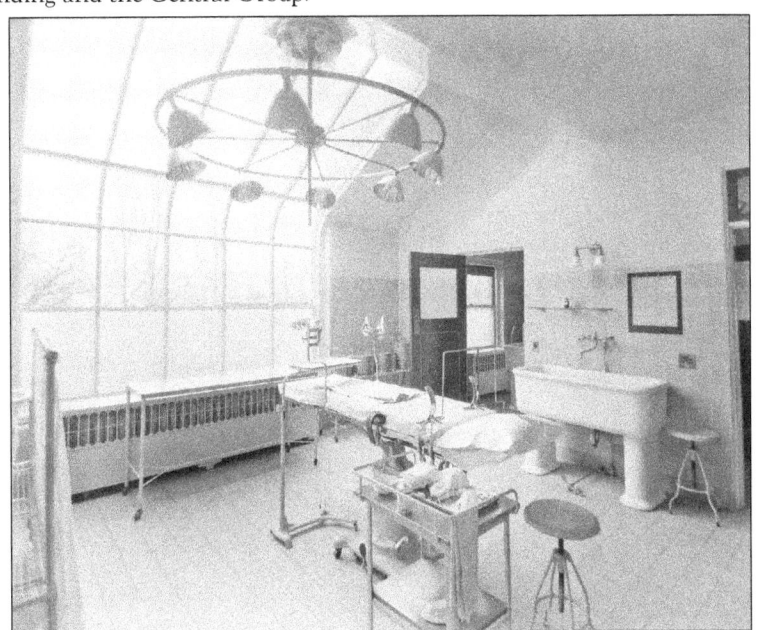

This was a state-of-the-art surgical suite in the early 1930s. Large glass panels were secured with airtight seals that did not open, in contrast to wooden sash windows. This was to promote a sterile environment. Patients and staff alike utilized the medical facilities at Hudson River.

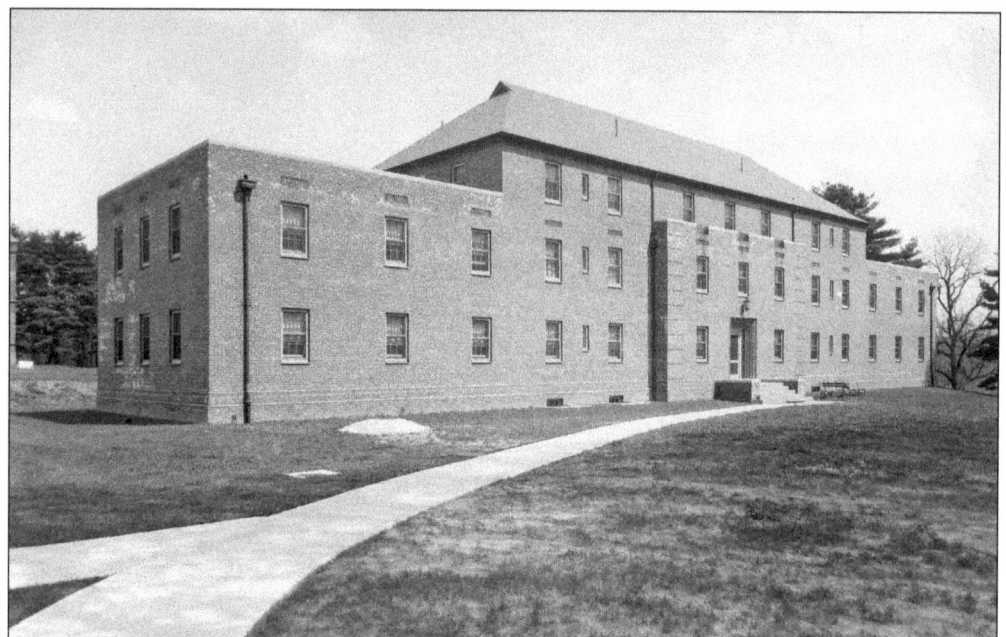

Buildings for patient housing were not the only construction projects to take place in the 20th century at Hudson River. No longer required to live on the grounds during the medial part of the century, many staff still enjoyed the luxury. Poucher Home, shown above, opened in 1934 for 25 married couples working at the hospital. In later years, it became student nurse housing.

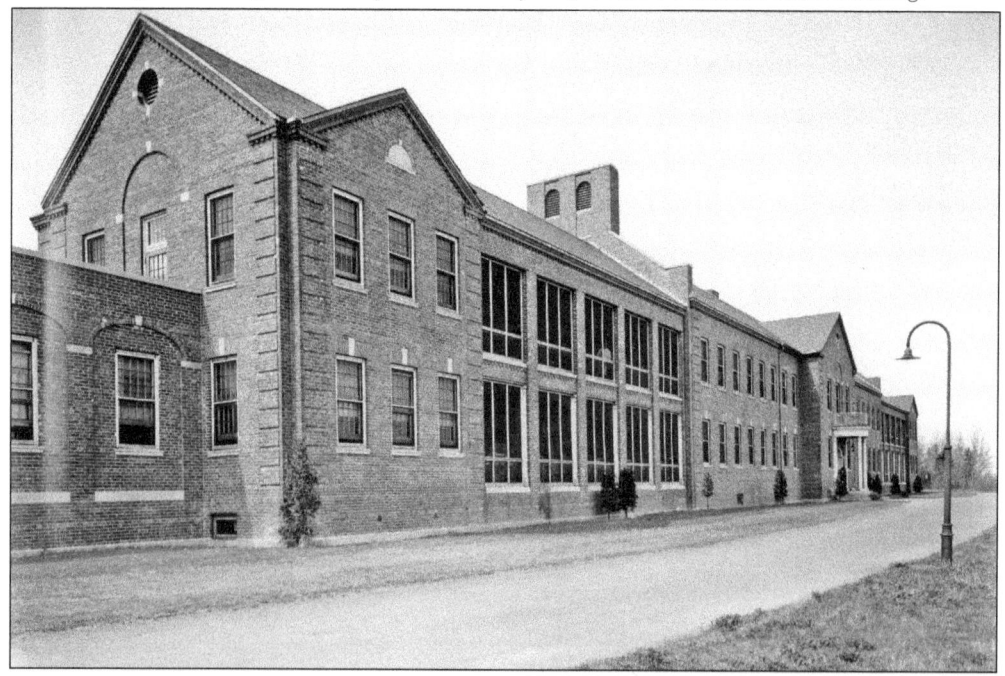

The first freestanding children's unit at Hudson River opened in 1934. Hillcrest School served children who required inpatient hospitalization for mental illness, while still providing a wholesome educational experience. This building's purpose changed over the decades. It is still operational today as a county homeless shelter.

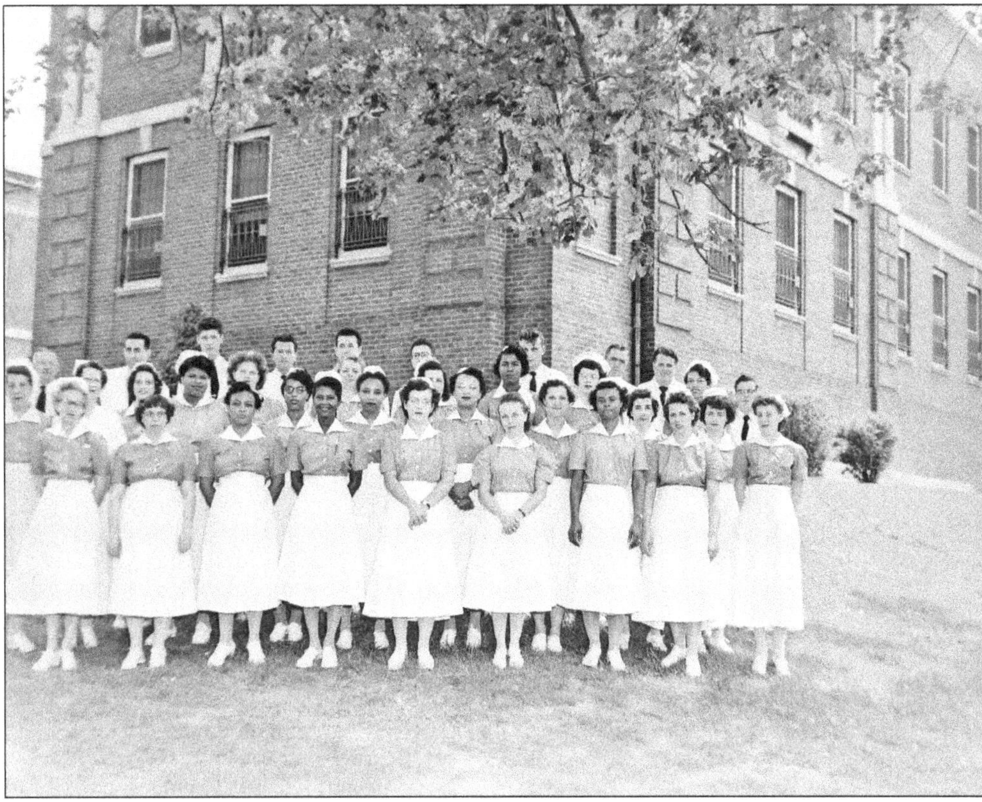

Ryon Hall opened in 1935 for additional space to house the soaring population of patients. Designed for 200 male and 200 female patients to be separated on identical wards to the east and west, Ryon Hall treated those who were in need of continuing care at Hudson River. This, in the addition to the opening of the nearby Harlem Valley State Hospital in Wingdale, New York, greatly combatted overcrowding. In this 1950s image, a newly graduated class of psychiatric aids poses for a photograph outside the building.

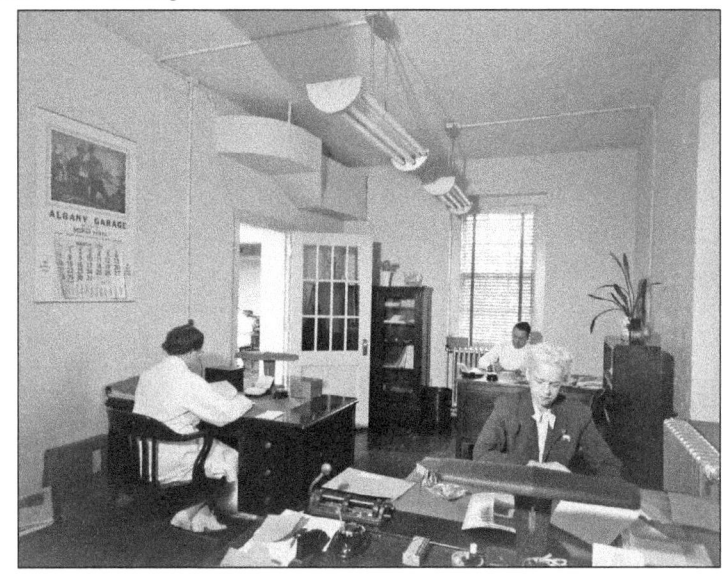

In addition to patient wards for men and women, Ryon Hall had a modern cooking school. If one took a walk downstairs to the school in 1954, this would have been the sight upon entry. Here, the central office for the school housed its secretary, instructors, and supervisors.

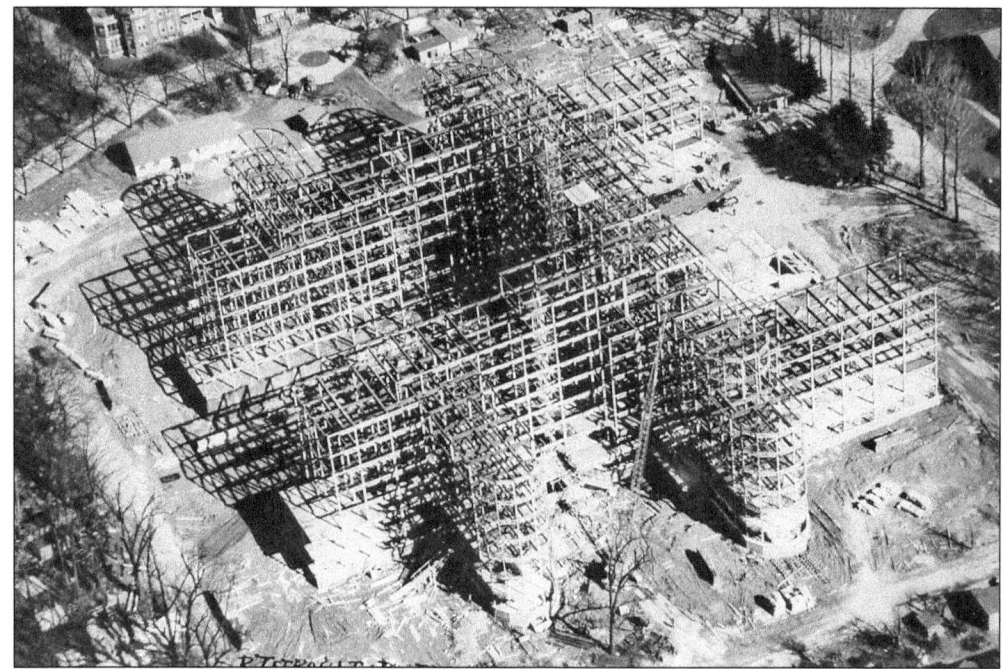

This aerial photograph was taken around 1950 and shows the steel skeleton of the Cheney Memorial building during its fabrication. This medical hospital building was the largest single structural project at Hudson River during the 20th century. Unlike many of its predecessors, Cheney was made entirely of steel with concrete floors, not wood, making its extremely durable and fireproof.

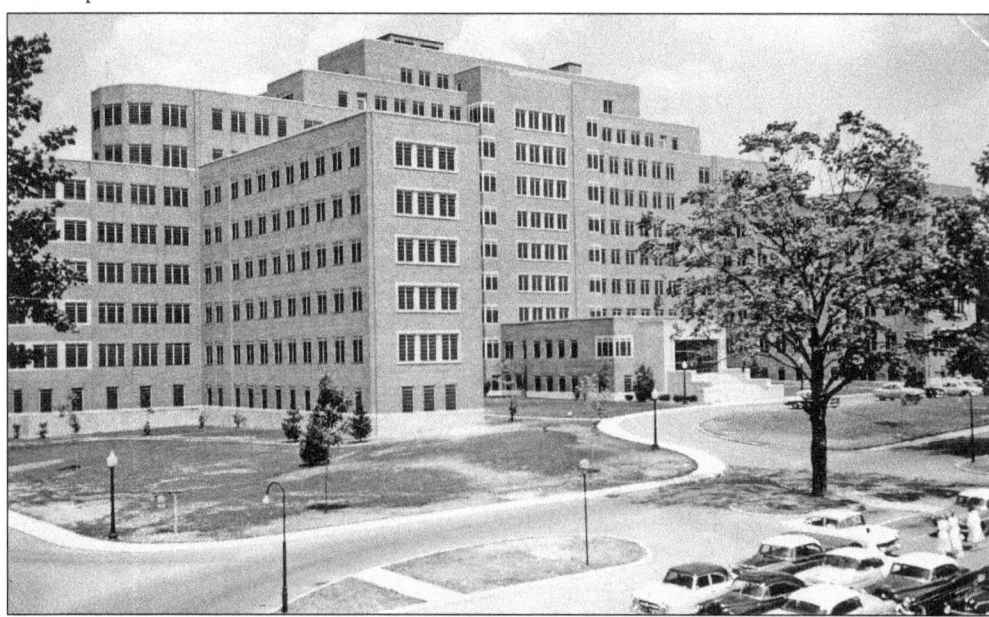

In 1949, construction on Cheney Memorial, named after director Clarence O. Cheney, was under way. This massive 960-bed medical hospital for Hudson River opened in 1952. It is incredible to think that the facility was so large that it needed its own medical hospital rivaling neighboring county hospitals in size. Though it was repurposed, Cheney Memorial remained open until 2001.

Just as buildings were needed to accommodate tradesmen in metal and carpentry shops, space for production by patient workers increased with the size of the facility. This 1951 image shows an extension off the back of the main building for occupational therapy. This could have been a number of production-based jobs, later called vocational rehabilitation.

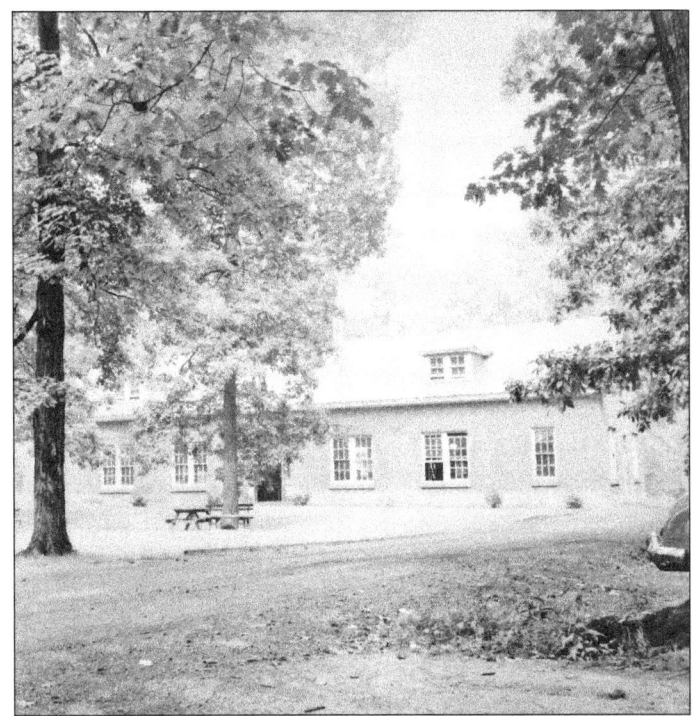

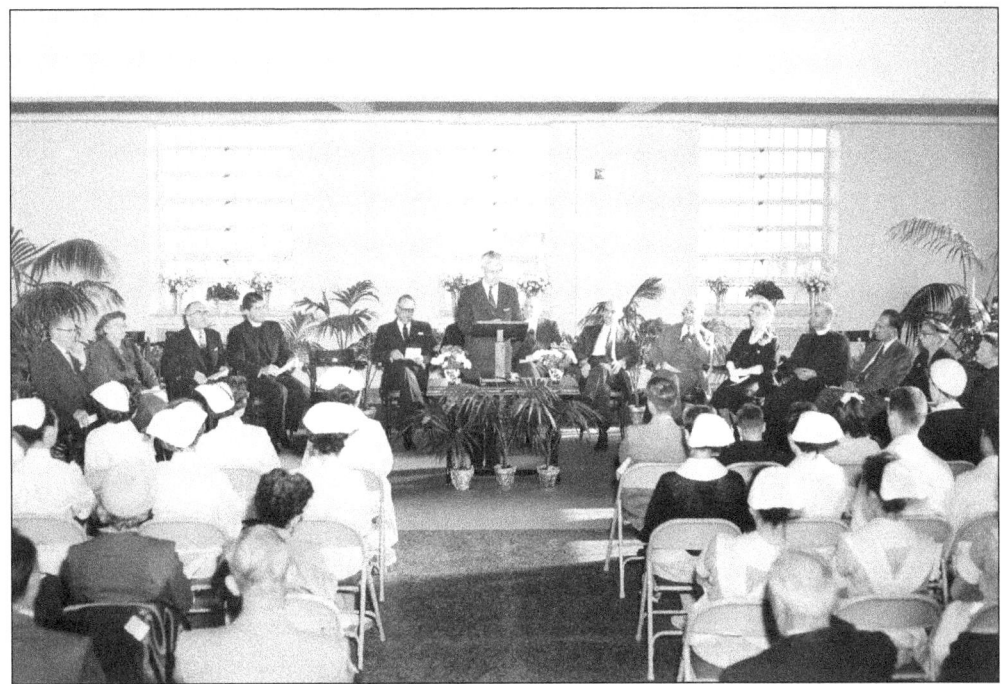

A new building opened in 1954 for the care of patients with active tuberculous; as TB was eradicated, this became a psychogeriatric building. On November 6, 1957, the building was dedicated to John Ross, MD, the sixth director of Hudson River. This image was taken during the dedication ceremony. Ross was renovated for the 2001 move to the "upper campus" and was the last building to house inpatients when the hospital closed on January 25, 2012.

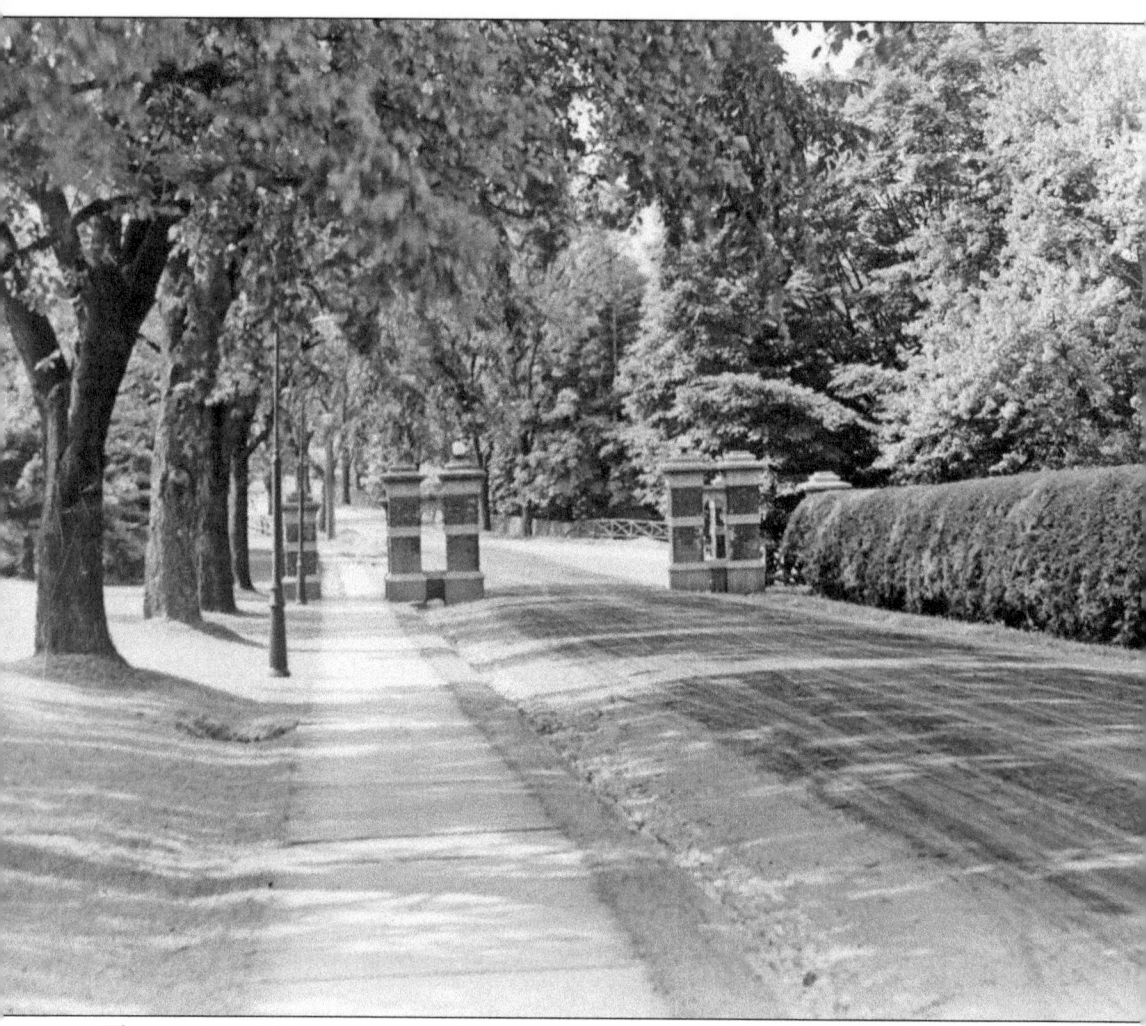

The remains of this once-proud brick entrance marker can still be found today off Route 9G in Poughkeepsie, just across from Marist College. This was the first sight individuals encountered upon entering the grounds of Hudson River State Hospital. On the street side, metal signs reading "Hudson River State Hospital" were affixed to the red brick. After passing these ornate markers, a long road heavily lined with trees wound in a snakelike bend up to the main building's heightened plateau. It was reminiscent of a drive through a park, not too surprising when considering the landscape was the work of Frederick Law Olmsted, the designer of Central Park in New York City. This photograph was taken with a view looking downhill at the rear of the brick pillars that marked the main entranceway heading back out to Route 9G.

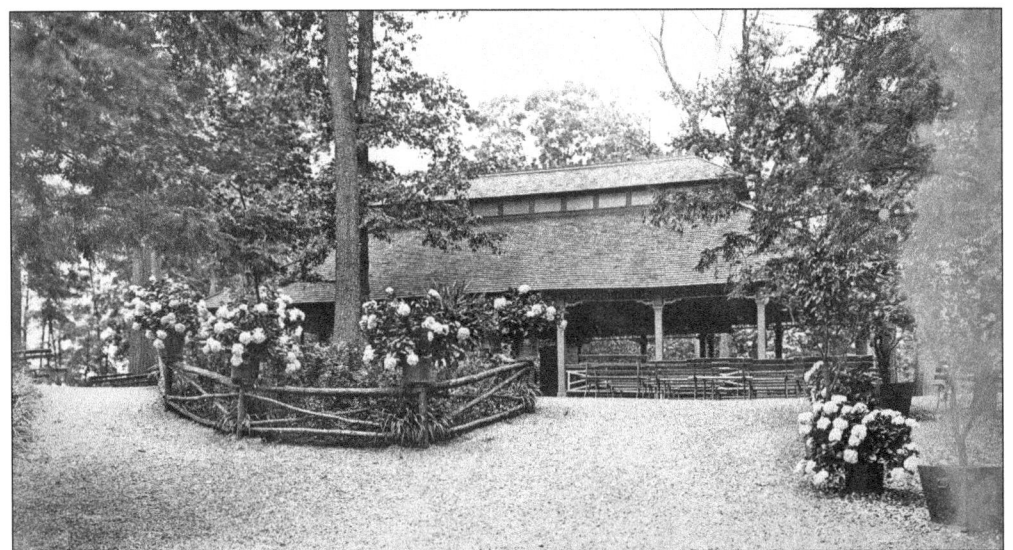

One of many constructed on the scenic grounds of the hospital, this pavilion surrounded by tall pines was for staff and patient social activity. A sense of tranquility and freedom could not help but be experienced, despite the setting of a psychiatric hospital. Outdoor activities were common and encouraged for all.

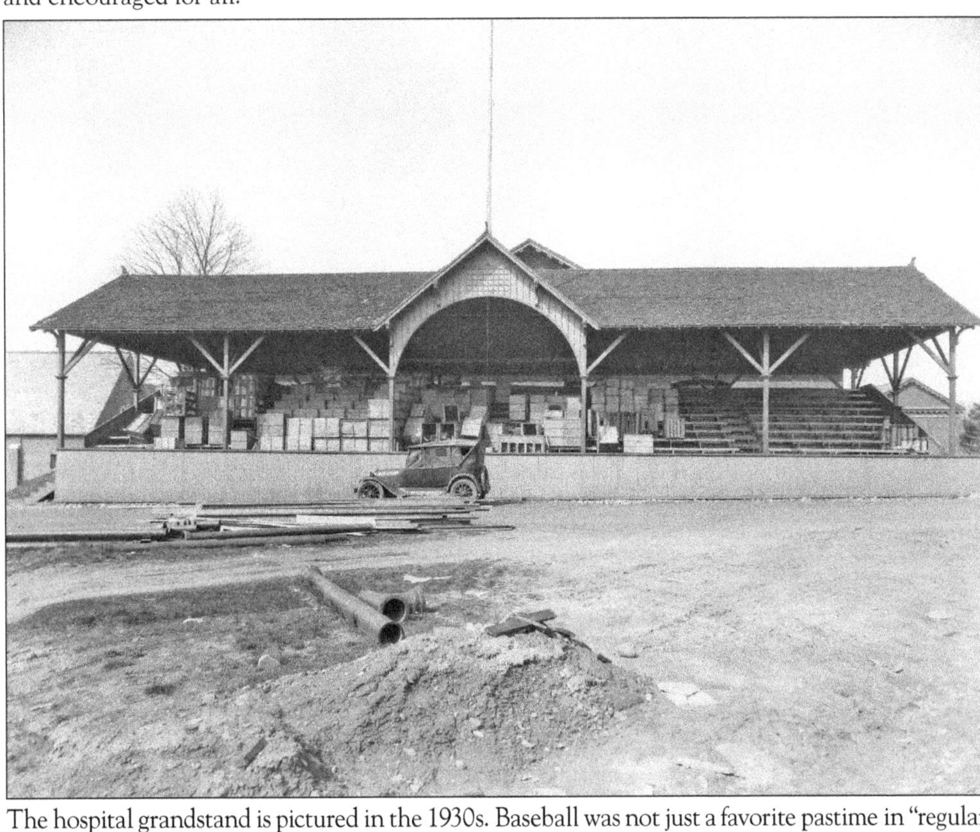

The hospital grandstand is pictured in the 1930s. Baseball was not just a favorite pastime in "regular" American life; at Hudson River, games were routinely held between staff, patients, and the state hospital league. This image shows construction work on a new men's ball field at the hospital.

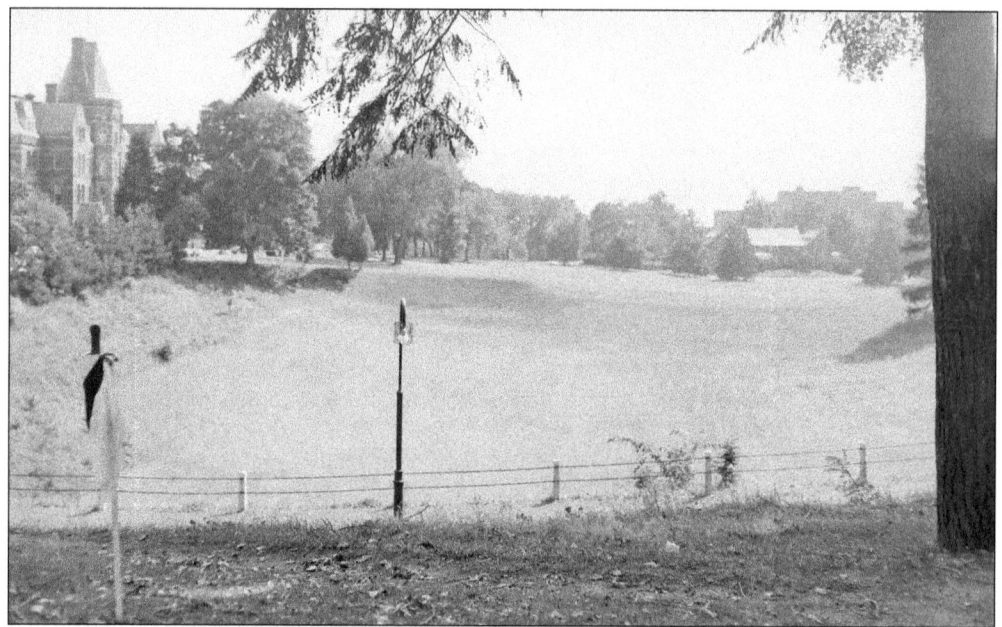

Hudson River was distinguished for several of its attractive grounds features, one being a sprawling golf course. The sloped, landscaped front lawn designed by Olmsted was converted into a golf course in the 1930s. This is a view from one of the golf holes; to the left, the main building's roof juts into sight. To the right, a silhouette of Cheney Memorial's roof can be seen.

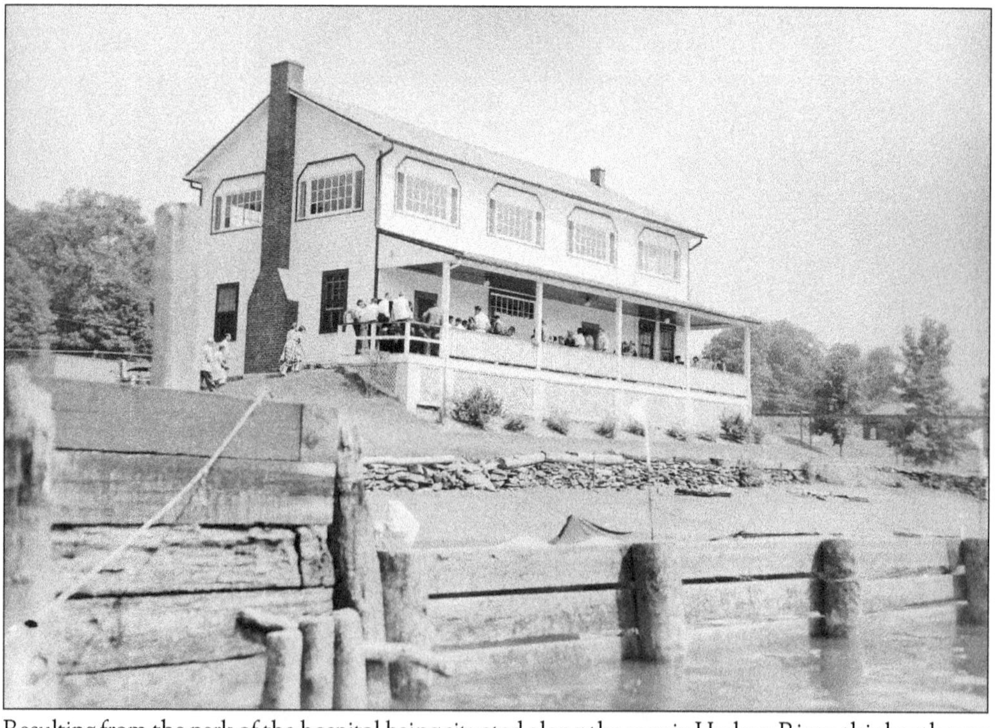

Resulting from the perk of the hospital being situated along the scenic Hudson River, this boathouse was constructed for patient recreational activity. Staff utilized this building as well, even chartering a boat club. This site was a favorite spot for summer social events at the hospital.

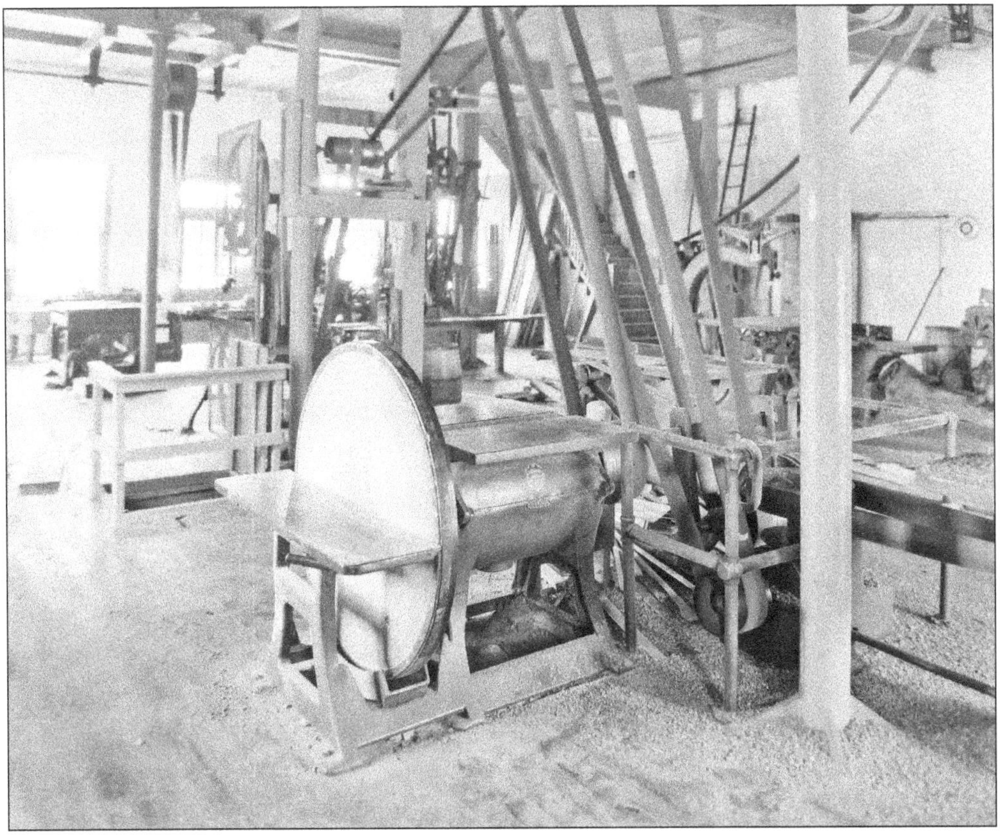

Before the conversion to electric machines, steam-powered shafts ran the length of many service buildings. Here, in the carpentry shop, the large belts that powered machines can be seen at rest. When the spindle on the ceiling was running, belts could be kicked on and off to operate the massive machines.

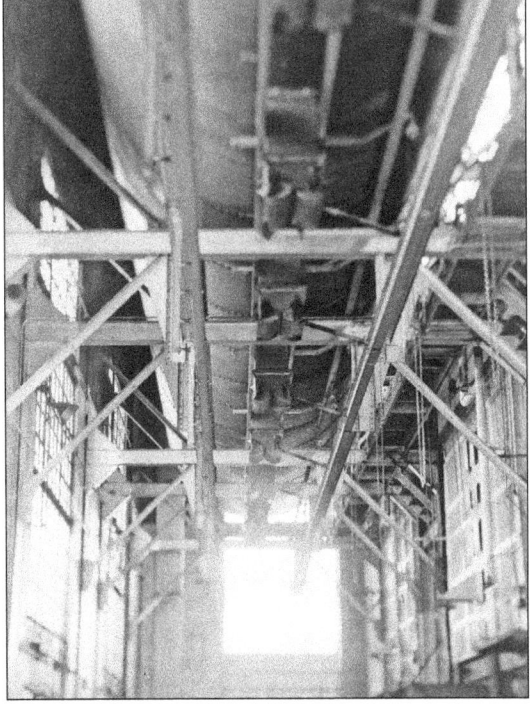

Coal remained the primary fuel the hospital used until the 1980s, when the power plant was converted to gas and oil. Depending on which fuel was cheaper that day, the boilers fired gas or oil respectively. This 1954 image shows the coal hoppers that fed the burners supplying heat, hot water, and power to the facility.

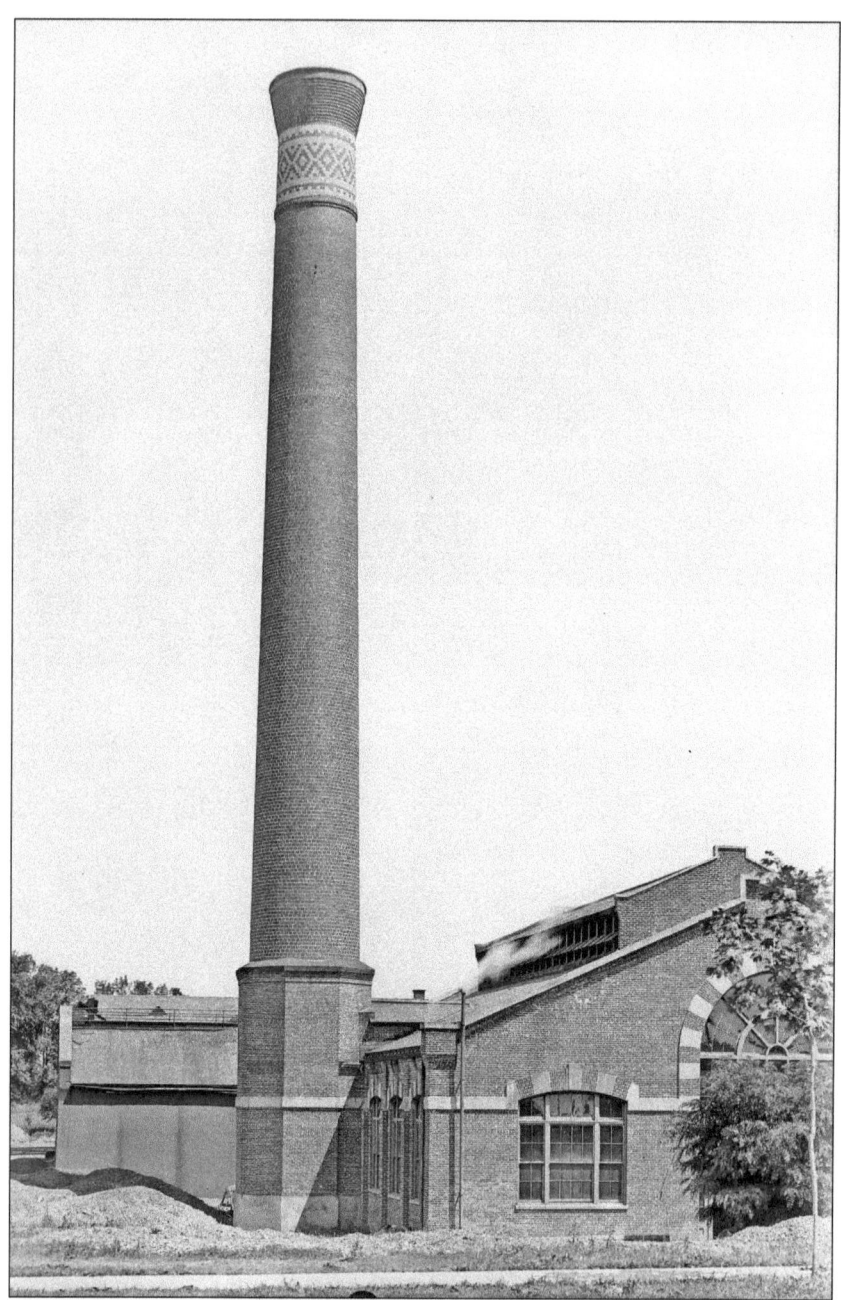

A power plant was an integral part of remaining an autonomous facility, which was the operating philosophy for many years. Hudson River was built decades before the advent of electricity, but it did initially have a generating plant to produce steam for heating and cooking. For obvious reasons, the hospital was quick to climb aboard modern times and construct a plant to generate its own electricity. Already having the mechanisms to produce steam made this economical, as electricity could be generated through the process that already was taking place. This smokestack belongs to an early power and boiler plant constructed to the rear of the main building. When the building opened, coal was burned to generate steam pressure. As time went on, the modern plant was retrofitted to burn oil and gas.

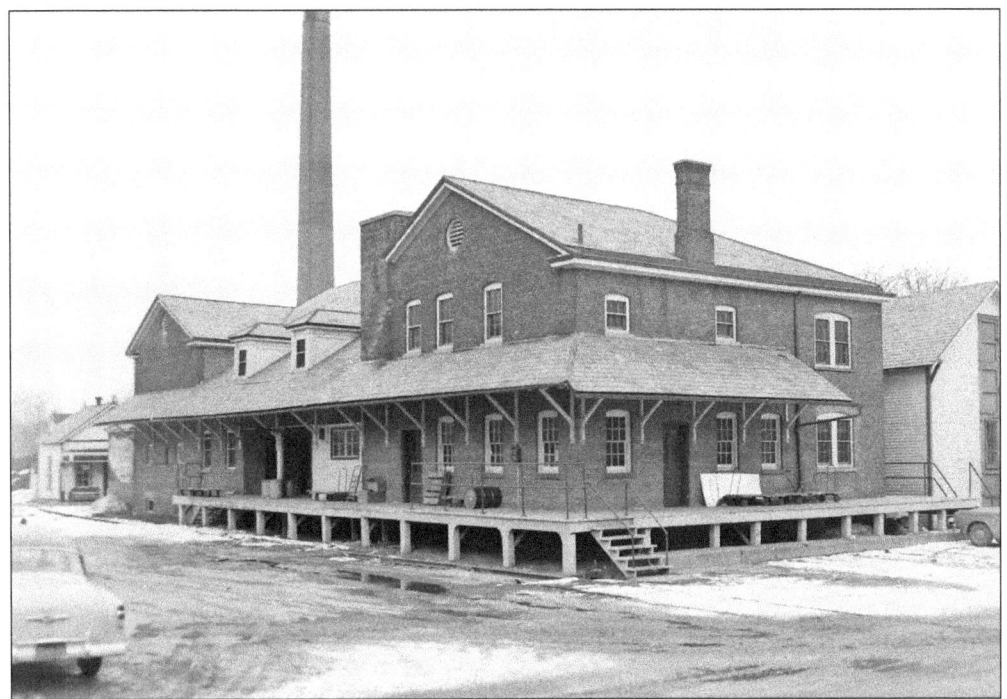

A building that is often overlooked but is perhaps one of the most critical to the hospital's operation was the storehouse. Almost every item that arrived at this hospital via mail, horse, car, or otherwise came here first for processing before delivery to the appropriate building. This 1954 photograph shows the loading dock on the storehouse where trucks would deliver goods.

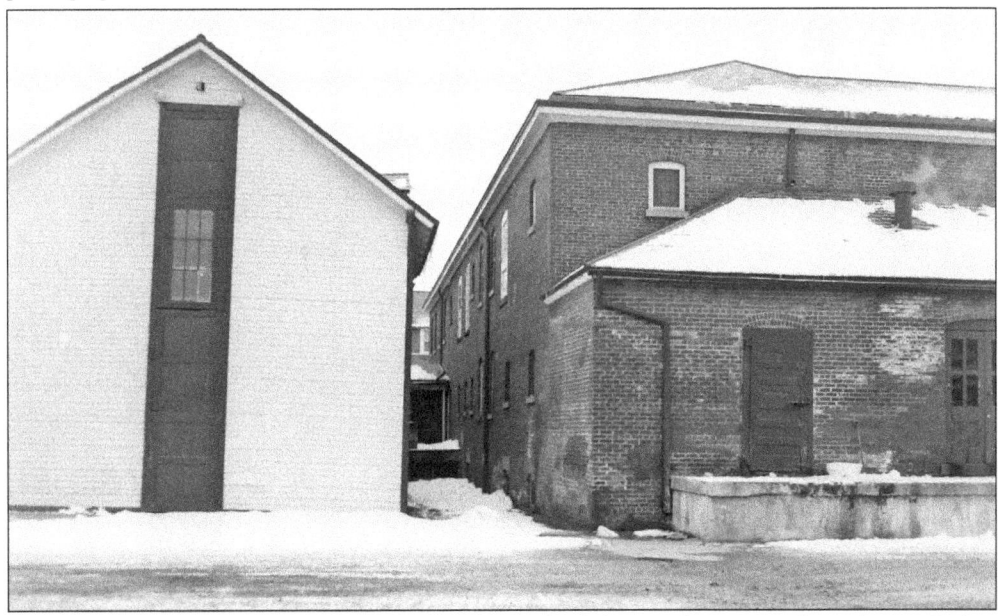

This white wooden structure added on to the east side of the storehouse was the icehouse. Before the advent of modern refrigerating systems, ice was harvested from a nearby creek and brought by horse and carriage for storage. Massive ice blocks were moved off the ground and up to the second-floor loft door via a lift system.

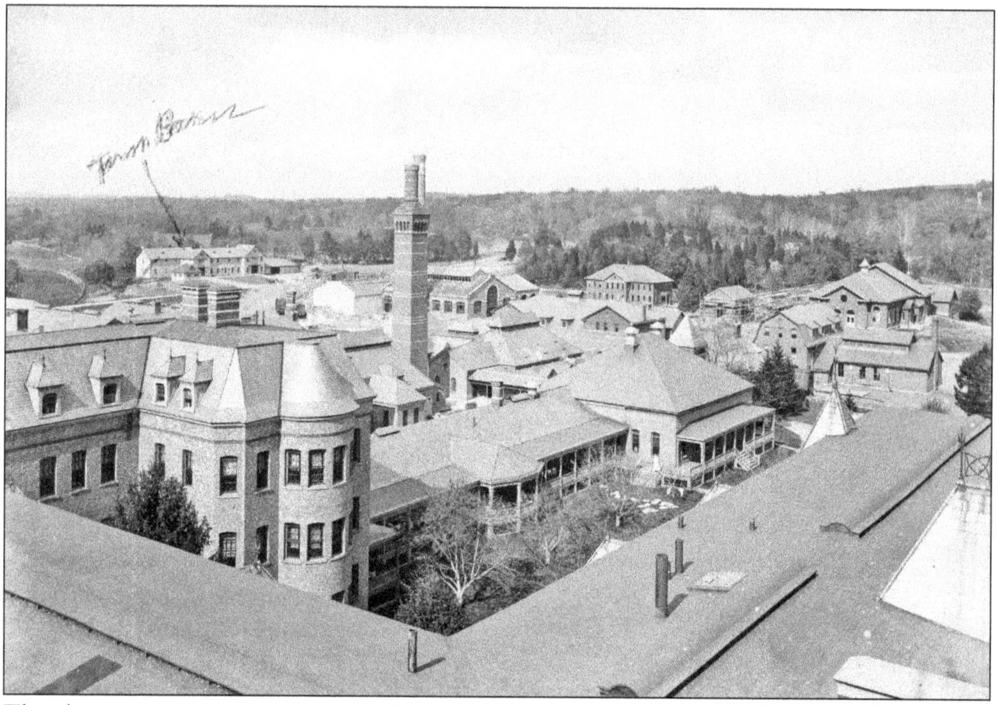

The above image was taken around 1910 from the roof of the main building; just about center frame, the patient library can be seen nearing completion. To the left, an arrow is drawn where the dairy farm existed. The photograph below was taken in 1906 during the construction of a cow barn at Hudson River. Here, the hospital raised and housed dozens of dairy cows. Excess milk was often taken to nearby state facilities in exchange for credit the steward could utilize in ordering other facilities' surplus food items, furniture, or sundries Hudson River needed. As the farms shut down, building purposes changed. Some barns were converted into storage sheds or even used as garages for cars.

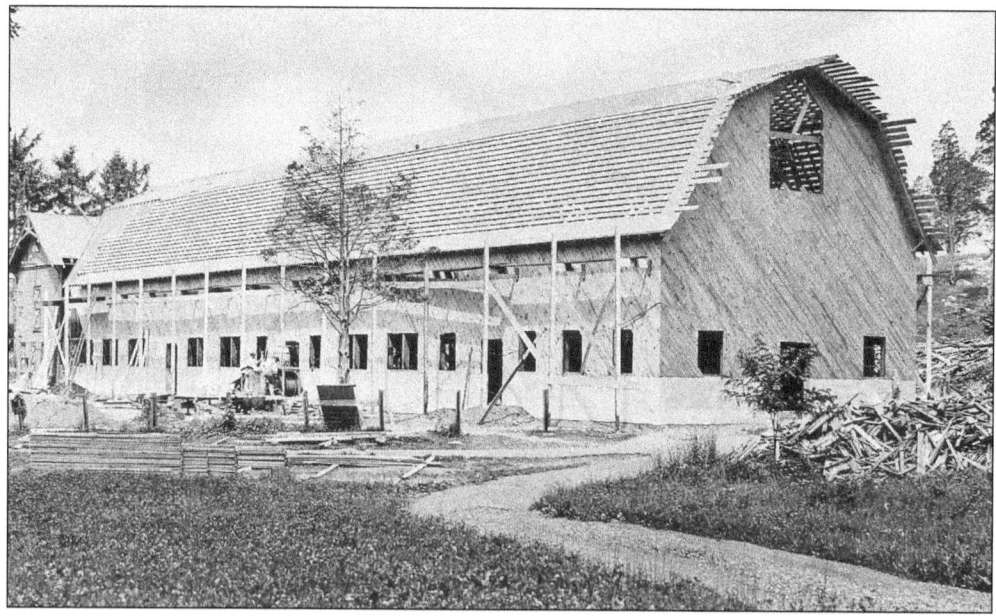

Two

Employee Life

Up until after World War II, attendants made up the majority of staff in the hospital; others who saw patients included nurses, doctors, and a few activities staff. The attendants worked under the license of a nurse and were responsible for duties including giving medication, counting patients, maintaining cleanliness of the wards, and providing 24-hour supervision of patients. Attendants worked 12-hour shifts, six days per week, and in 1935, their pay was $54 per month. Before the construction of separate staff quarters, many lived on the wards, with the patients in separate hallways. Fringe benefits supplemented the pay. Staff were provided room and board, meals, medical and surgical care if they ever required such, and uniforms. Every ward initially had its own dining room where both staff and patients would eat meals, often together. All staff wore uniforms until the 1970s. For male attendants, a white shirt, black tie, black shoes, and navy-blue pants and vest were required. Women attendants wore a blue uniform with a white bib apron and white cap. Improper dress was not an uncommon reason to be sent off duty without pay.

Written permission had to be granted for night personnel to go off grounds, as they were required to be on duty at 6:30 p.m. Night-shift attendants were required to check each individual patient every hour and record this through a punch clock. Day employees were required to be in bed without light by 11:00 p.m. and also were monitored by a watchman. It was not uncommon for staff to find creative ways to sneak out at night for a walk or a drink. Every employee was assigned a pass key, and losing one's keys was close to, if not, grounds for dismissal. Many of the founding staff were immigrants; advertisements in Irish newspapers encouraged people to migrate to America for work in the state hospitals. As a result, generations would work at Hudson River and other state facilities around the country.

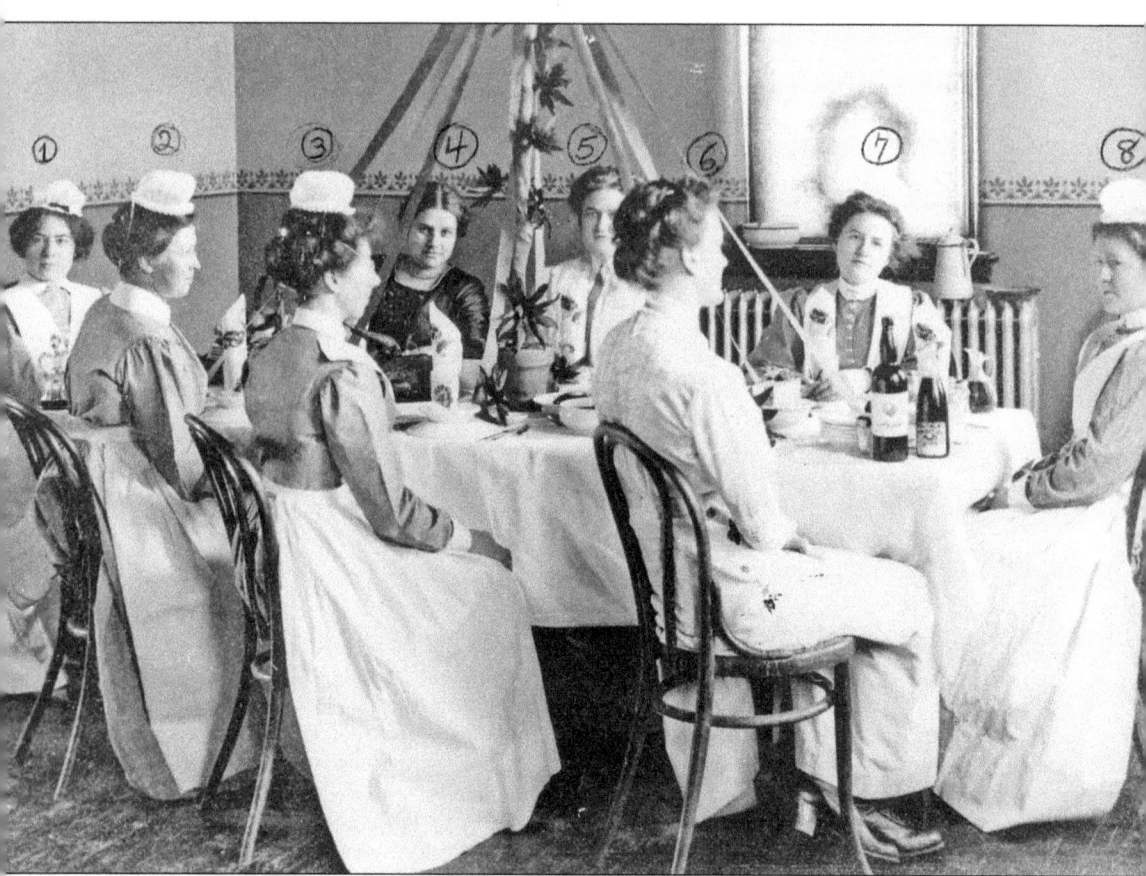

Like any other hospital facility, state psychiatric hospitals were in operation 24 hours a day, seven days a week. In order to keep the place running, it was often difficult to accommodate a large number of staff requests for time off during holidays. Instead, because of the greater hours required, holidays were often celebrated communally at work. This 1911 photograph taken in the main building shows the staff sitting down to Christmas dinner, presumably in the north wing, as fraternizing between sexes was not permitted at this time. Nurses and attendants would take turns preforming duties on the wards in order to allow other staff to eat a meal and socialize. Many off-hours ward staff would often celebrate with sweets for patients to enjoy and socialize even after a day of celebration provided by activities staff.

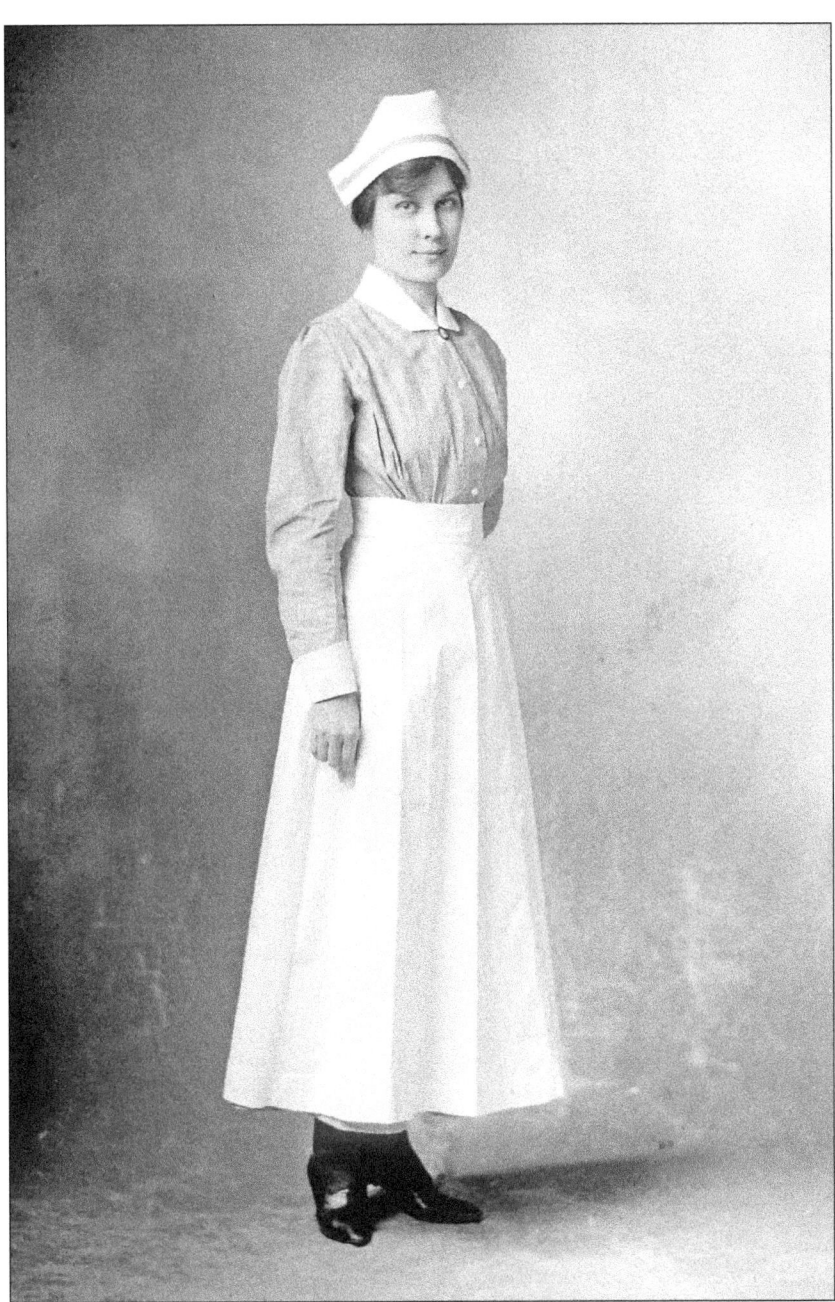

Employee uniforms were taken quite seriously in the earlier days of the hospital. Any man or woman not in regulation uniform would be sent off duty without pay. Men and women had their own dress codes. Both wore quite modest uniforms, with long selves and long dresses below the knees. The uniforms female nurses and attendants wore were very similar. In later years, it became easier to distinguish between the two by the number of stripes on their caps. In this 1918 picture taken in the photography studio of the main building, a female attendant poses in her hospital uniform. It was taken by the hospital photographer for use in a report to the managers regarding uniforms. In later years, attendants would become known as mental health therapy aides, commonly referred to as TAs.

Christmas was always celebrated on a grand scale at Hudson River. This 1970s photograph taken in the Snow Rehabilitation Center shows a staff member dressed up as Santa along with coworkers and patients singing carols in the center of the building for all to enjoy. As many patients were without family who visited, this could be an especially sad time of year if not for all the special attention on community celebration.

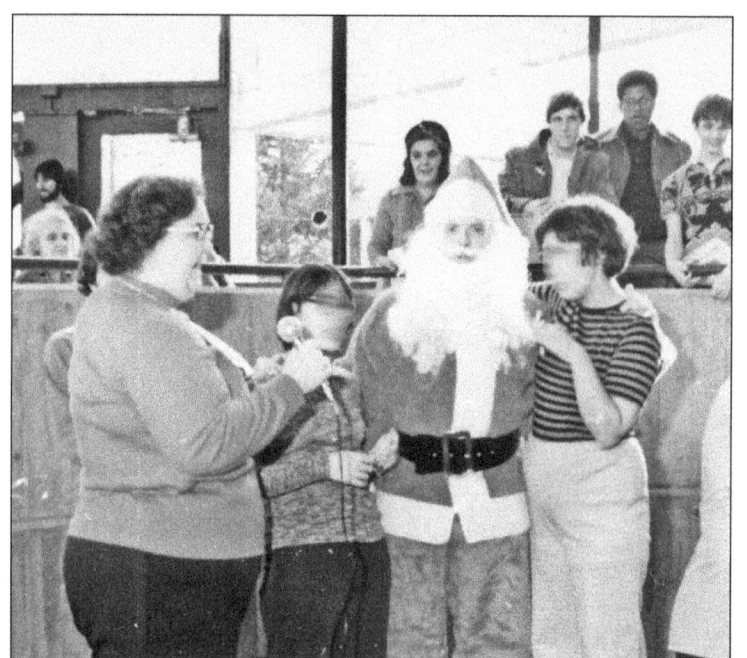

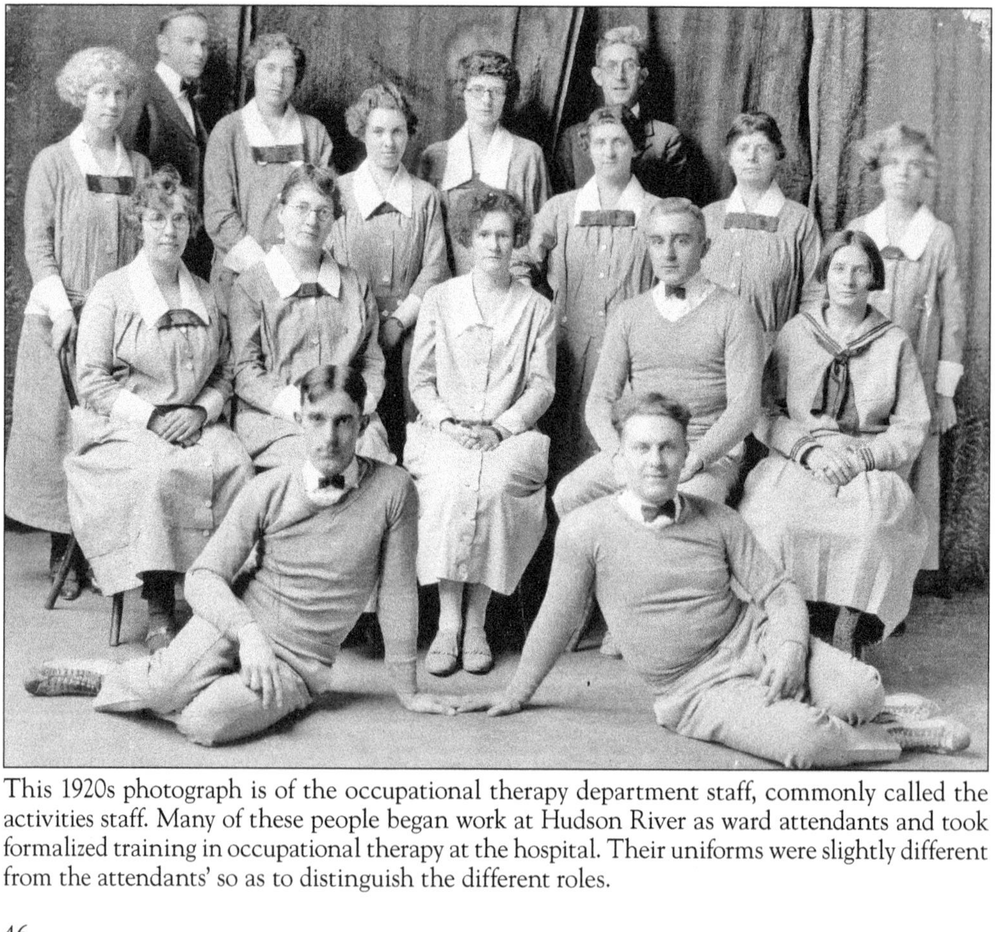

This 1920s photograph is of the occupational therapy department staff, commonly called the activities staff. Many of these people began work at Hudson River as ward attendants and took formalized training in occupational therapy at the hospital. Their uniforms were slightly different from the attendants' so as to distinguish the different roles.

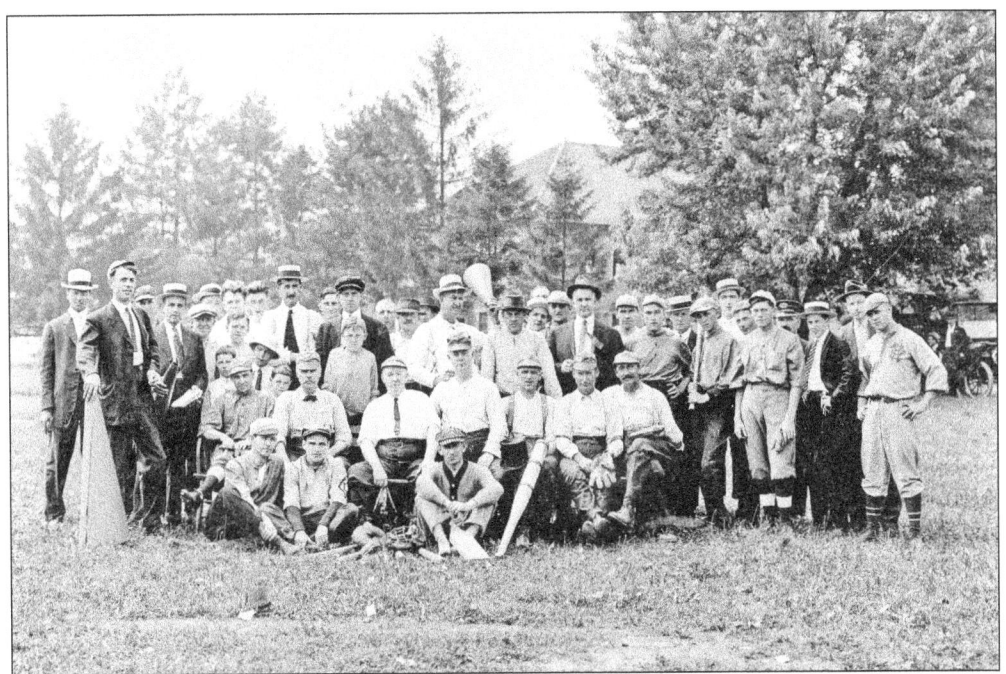

A little healthy completion between departments at the hospital always existed. This 1920s photograph is of the baseball team at Hudson River. Baseball was perhaps the most popular sport at this time at the hospital. Many teams were formed and competed against other state hospitals.

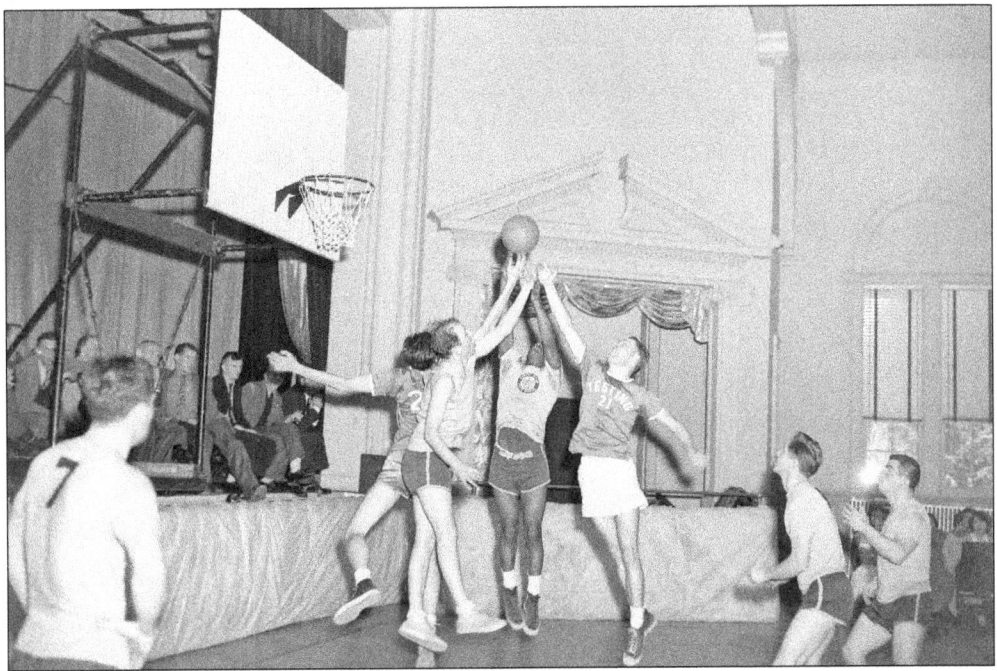

In the spirit of accepting a challenge, male staff at the hospital play a game of basketball against IBM workers in the Assembly Hall in 1954. This is another example of an opportunity to form a socially conjoined way of working and living among staff at Hudson River.

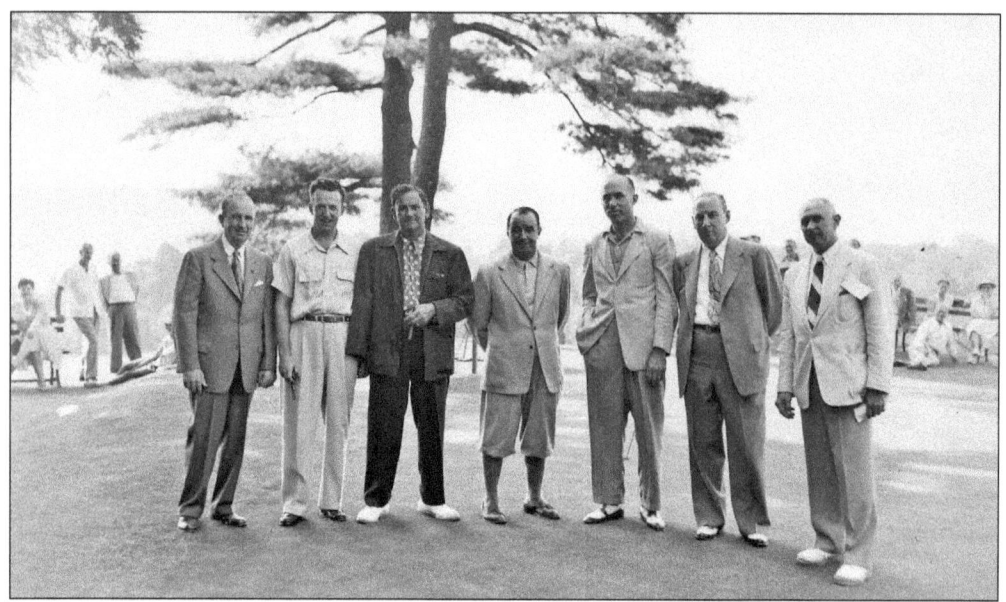

Another popular activity for all those who resided at Hudson River was playing on the upscale golf course. This group of men in 1952 is made up of staffers who made up the golf club. Clubs were a great way for staff to make friends with similar interests from various departments. This all added to a culture of family and pride at Hudson River.

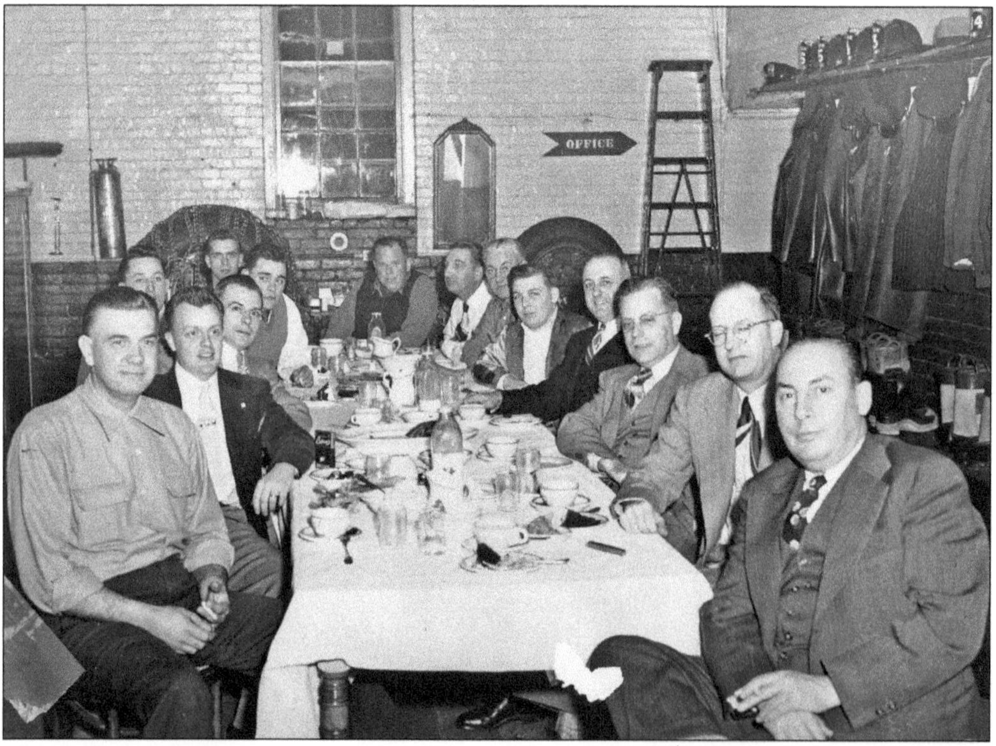

The ward personnel were not the only ones at the hospital to staff the facility at all times. This 1950s photograph was taken at the hospital's fire department. Communal meals were a common sight during this time, as many of the firemen were on watch for long shifts together.

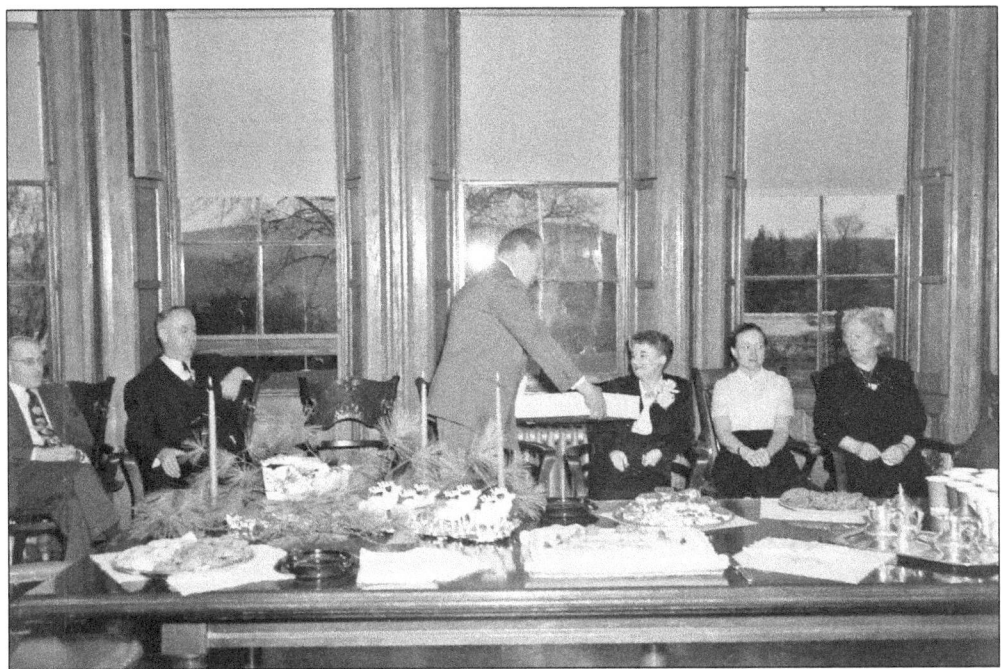

Retirements at Hudson River were bittersweet memories for many. While many were happy to start a new phase of life, they were often sad to give up their coworkers at the hospital, who became as close or closer than family. This 1950s image was taken in the administration building showing the retirement of a secretary working in the business office.

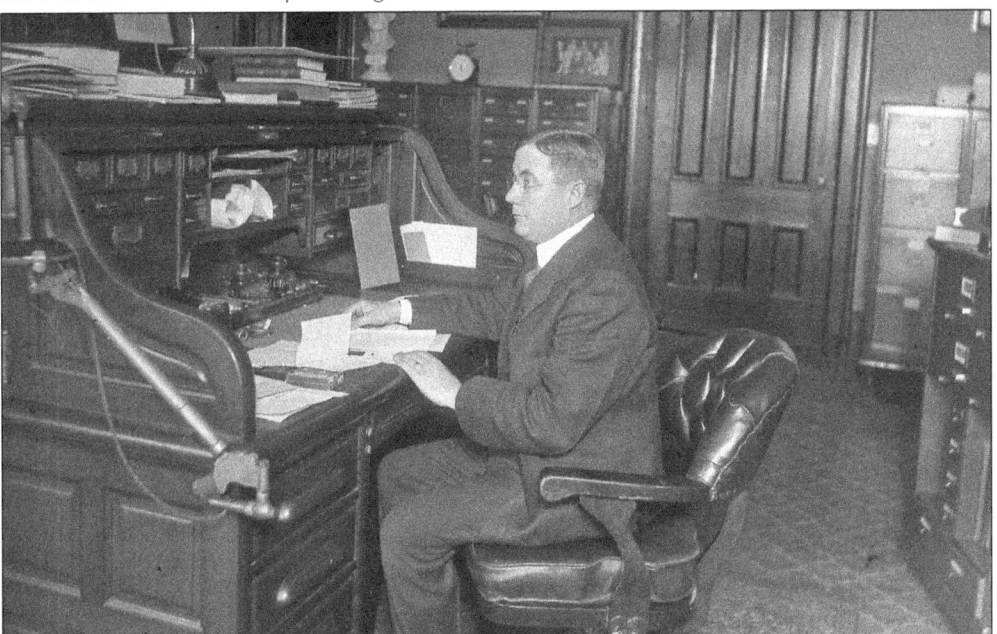

This photograph of the hospital steward around the turn of the century was taken in center building. The hospital steward was essentially the business manager of the facility, handling financial and budgetary matters. Gentlemen such as this worked eight-hour days and could live in private arrangements on the hospital grounds.

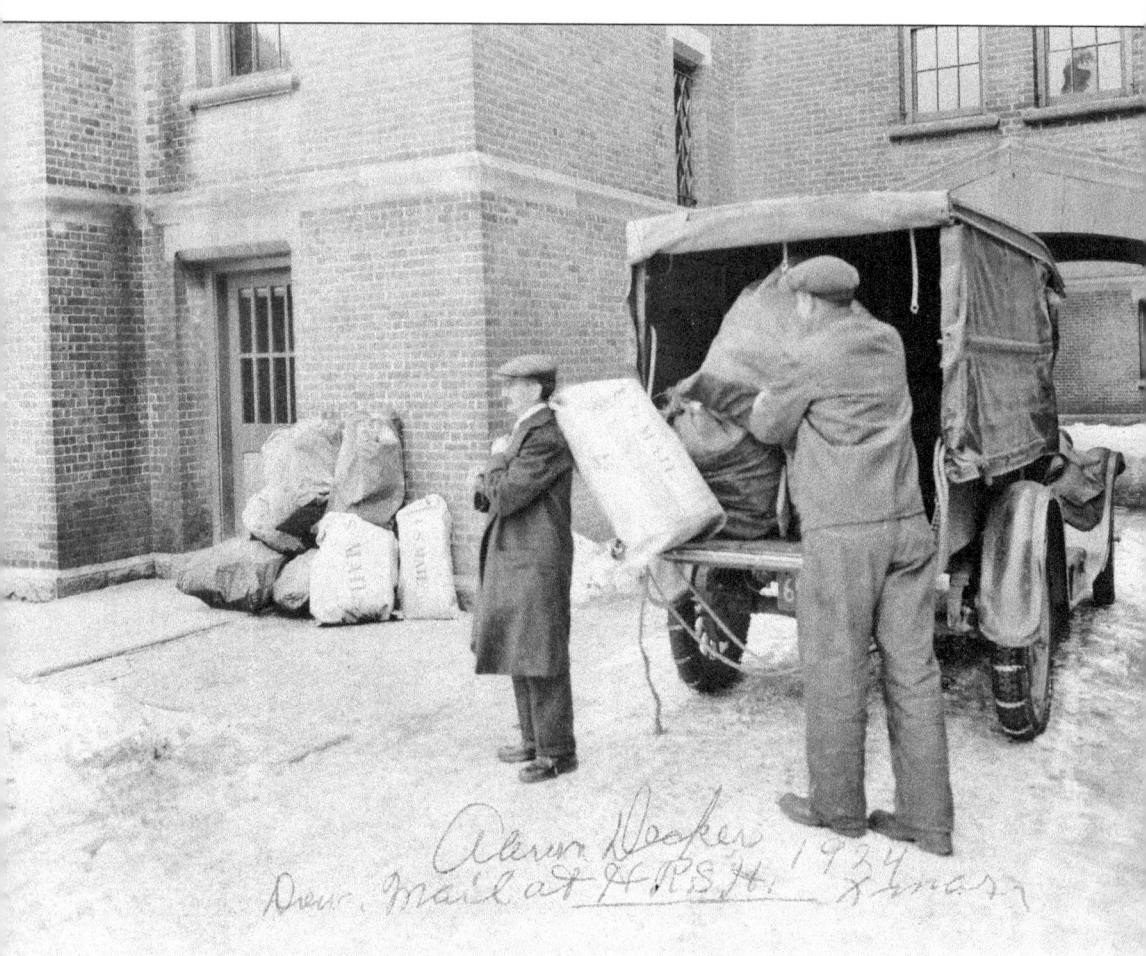

Mail was delivered to a central location at the storehouse then distributed through the hospital by staff from that department. It was loaded into vehicles for delivery around the grounds to all the buildings. Just like that of a US postman, this was an all-day job, since there were many buildings to deliver mail to and from. This 1924 photograph shows a mail delivery truck driven by A. Deaker pulling up to the main building on Christmas. Awaiting mail was undoubtedly an important part of the day for many patients who lived at Hudson River. At this time, writing and receiving letters or postcards were the primary means of communication between patients and outside friends or family. Eagerly awaiting gifts from loved ones on the holidays made the sight of the mail truck a happy one for many.

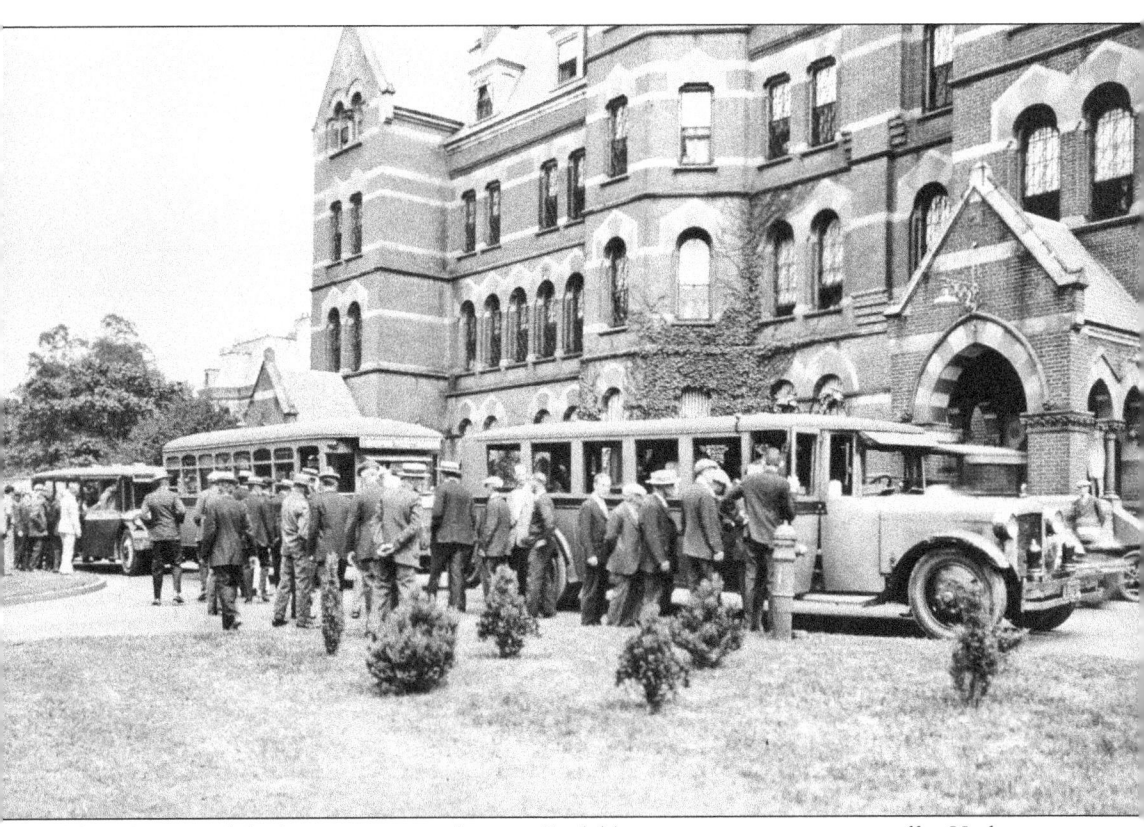

Although automobiles became more and more affordable as time went on, many staff at Hudson River earned a modest wage that could not support that purchase. Resultant from early operating policies, most of the staff historically lived on grounds. Because of the room and board with a modest wage, there was no real drive for many staff to pursue cars in the earlier 20th century. When staff training was held at other facilities, Hudson River would provide transport to those events. If staff got together in large enough numbers occasionally—for example to see a baseball game in New York City—this also was something for which transportation was provided from time to time. This 1930s photograph, taken outside of the administration building, shows the male staff of the hospital loading into a car and trolley for a trip. In the front at right, a hospital policeman can be partially seen near the portico of the building.

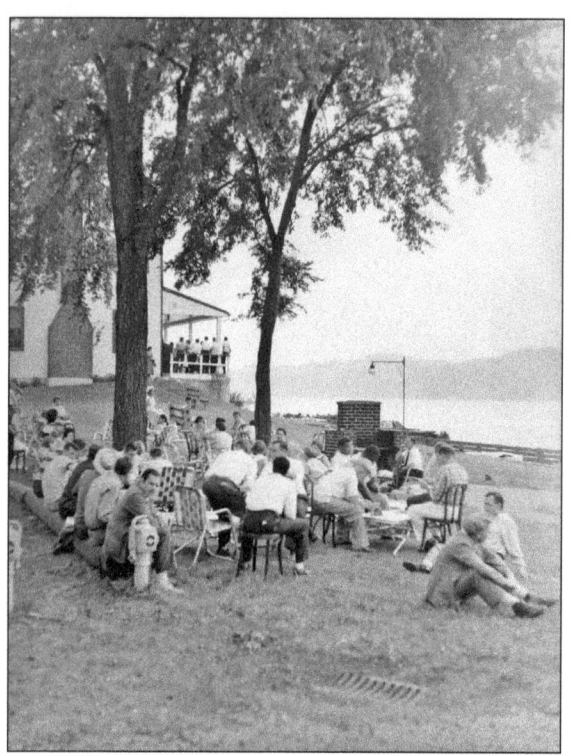

This 1940s photograph shows the boathouse in the spring. The staff are having a social event here. Facilities like this were open to all staff who wished to use them, even for family events. It would appear the porch facing the Hudson River was a popular spot to gather.

This scene is almost from a classic movie. Looking out the windows of the hospital boathouse is an excited group of young nurses. They are awaiting the arrival of Gov. Nelson Rockefeller for lunch and a tour of the hospital. Surrounding the governor, New York State Police officers don their class A dress uniforms.

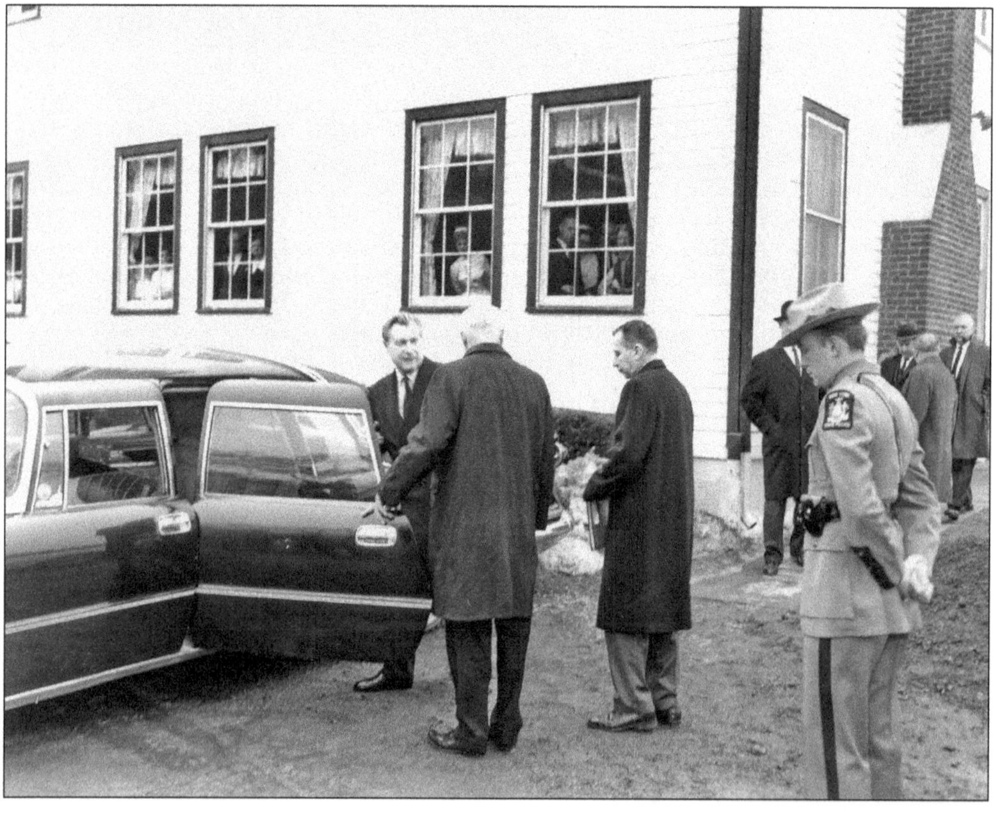

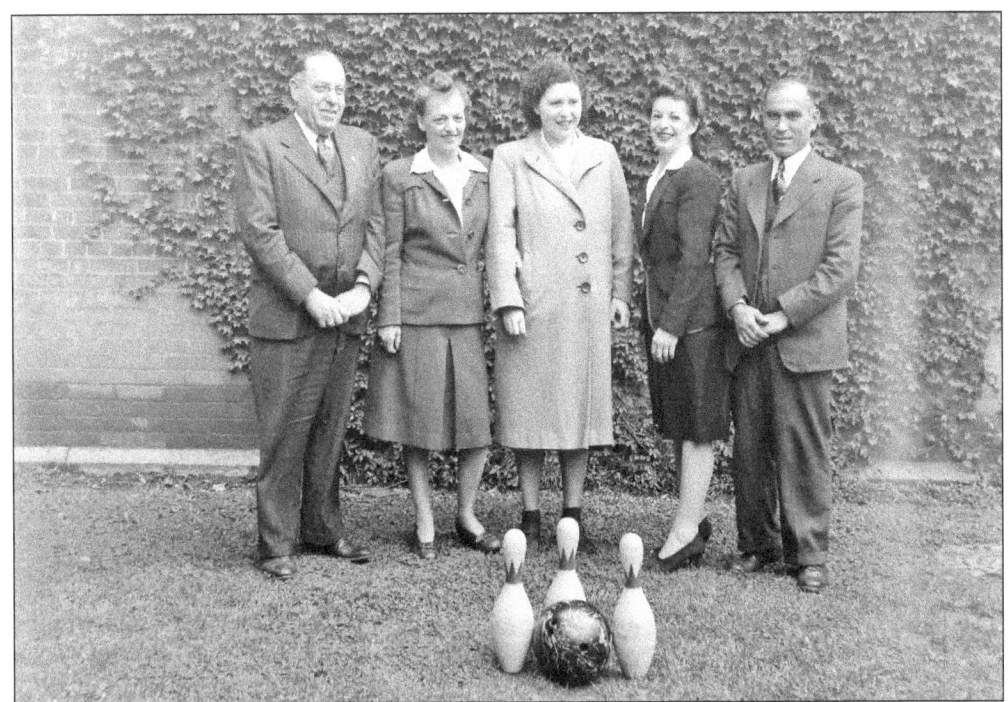

This 1951 image shows of the hospital's bowling team. In the 1950s, bowling was a very popular activity at Hudson River and the rest of the country. This was one of the few team sports at the hospital where men and women were not separated by sex in competition.

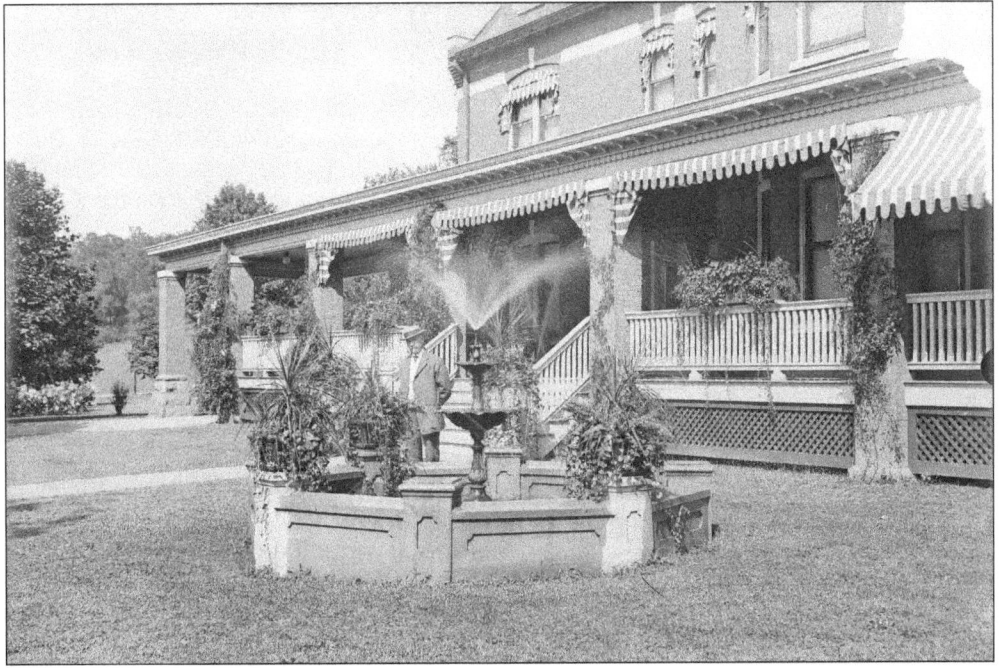

A man stands by the fountain outside the superintendent's mansion around 1918. He is presumably a farmer, judging by the type of hat he wears. This image, taken in the spring, shows the ornamental gardening that staff and patients would work together on at the hospital.

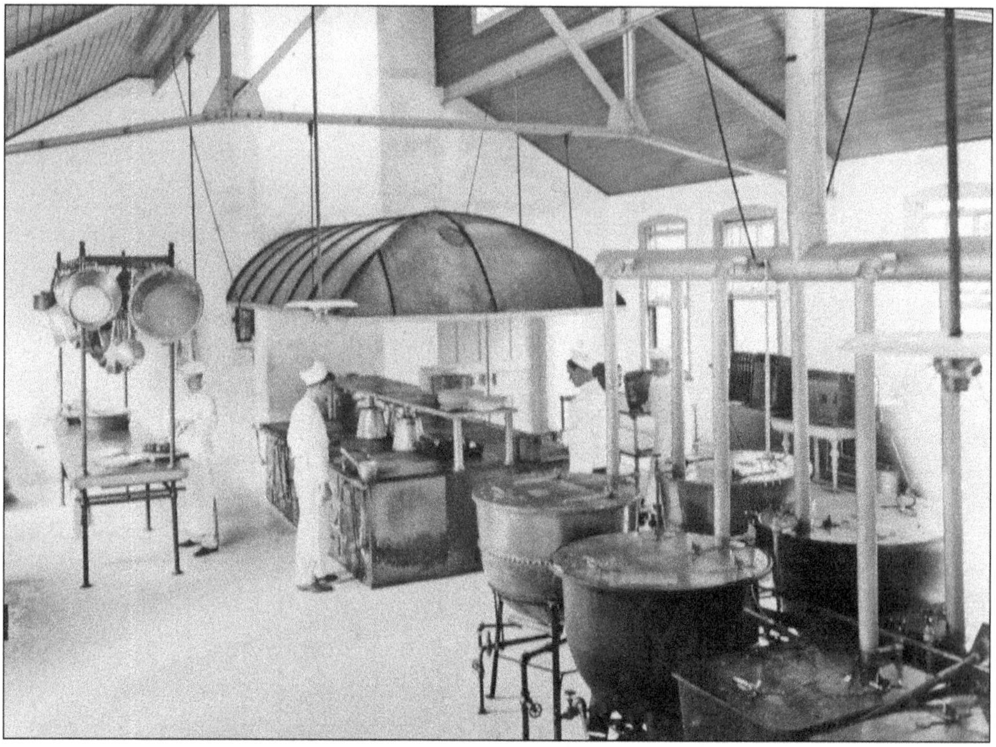

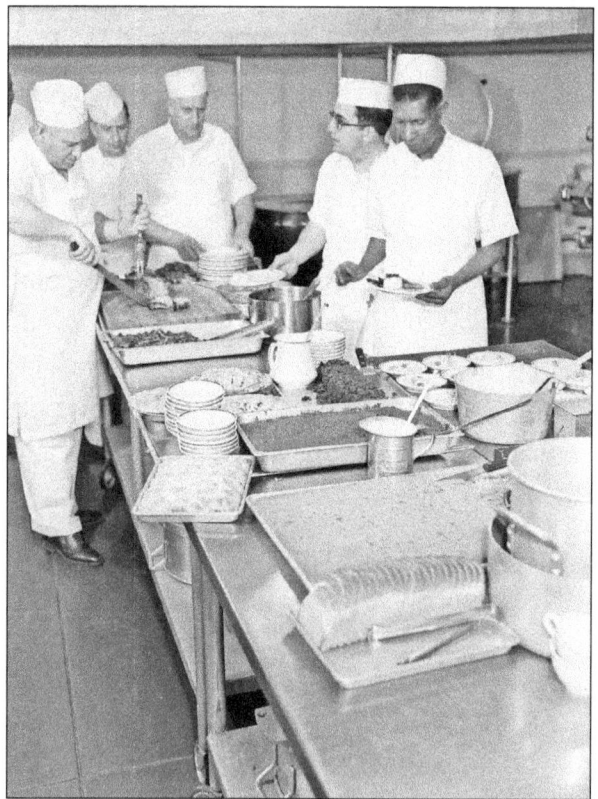

All meals were prepared entirely at the hospital until the late 1990s. This image, taken in the kitchen of the main building in the late 19th century, shows the steam-powered caldrons and large ovens needed to prepare hundreds of meals a day. Food service staff were also required to wear a uniform, all white, as can be seen here.

Attention to detail and quality was not restricted to medical and psychiatric services at Hudson River. This 1940s image was taken at the hospital's food service training school. Meals were served family style until the 1990s—large pans of food were dished out by staff. Often there was enough for seconds. This image shows one of the students tasting a meal.

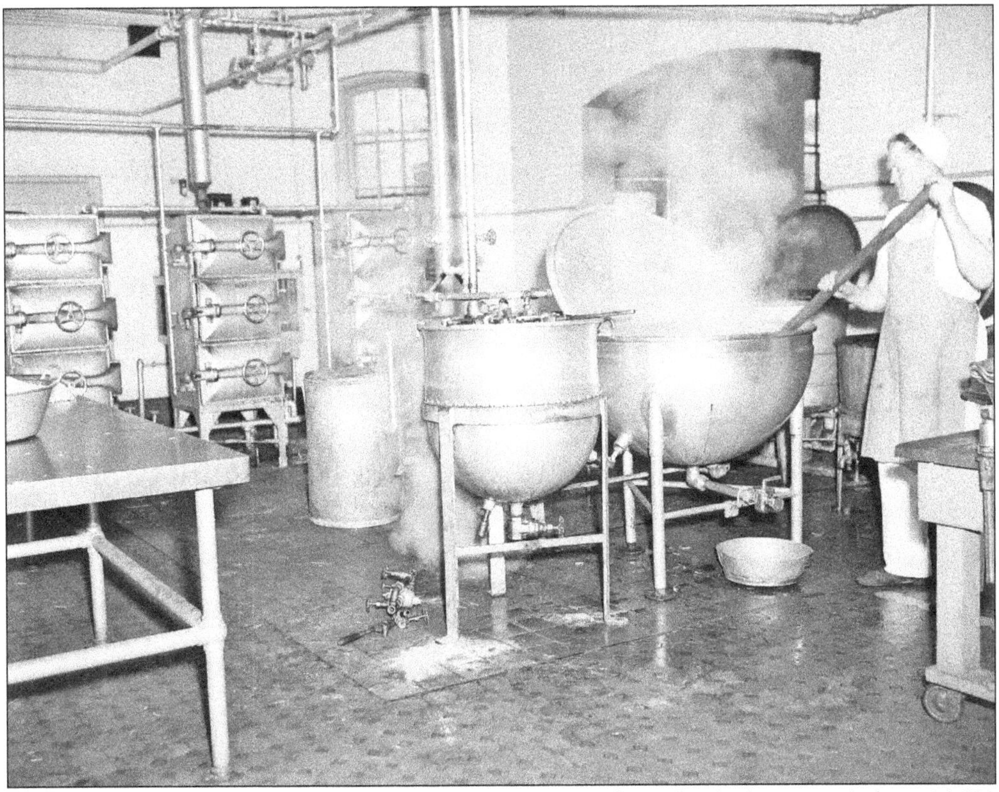

With around 5,500 patients at the time this image was taken, the facility served about 16,500 meals daily. Preparing that volume of food does not leave much room for broken equipment. This photograph, taken on July 26, 1951, shows a food service worker preparing soup faithfully while a broken pressure cooker leaks hot steam on his left, awaiting repair.

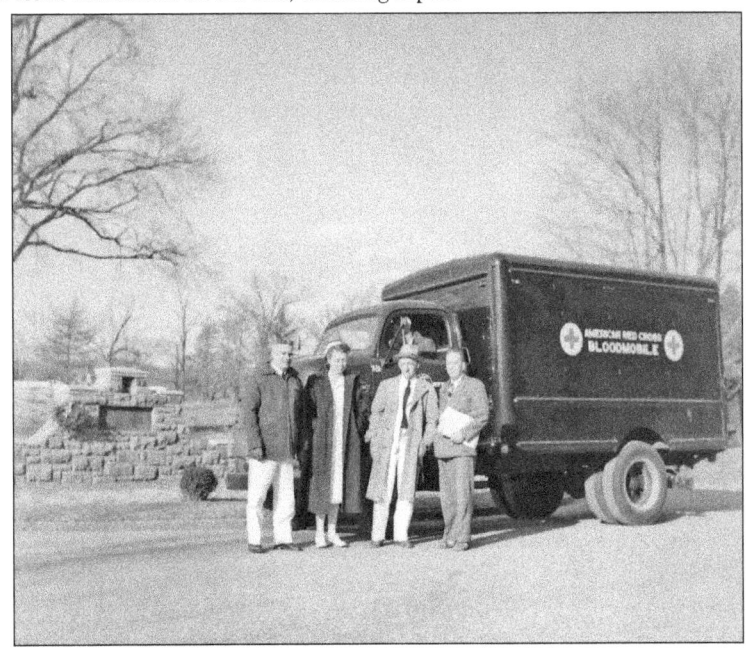

This 1952 photograph shows a truck transporting all the supplies needed to set up a mobile blood drive at Hudson River or anywhere else. At the time, in exchange for their donation, staff could get a few hours off duty or small rewards from the blood-collecting agency.

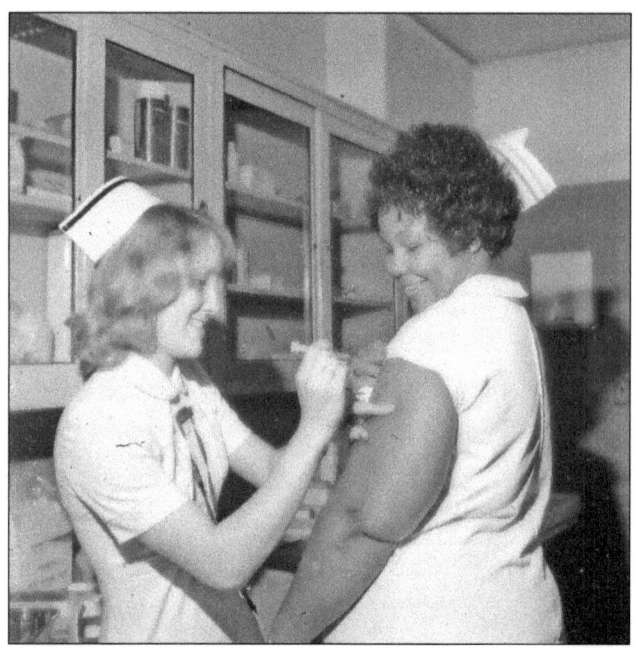

Employee health was a concern of the facility, since in any hospital setting, minimizing the chances of spreading illness is imperative. In addition to yearly checks for tuberculosis, staff underwent yearly vaccines to prevent diseases. This photograph, taken in November 1976, showcases a recently graduated student nurse from the hospital's training school. The author of this book and an employee at Hudson River for 22 years, Lynn Rightmyer, RN, gives out a swine flu vaccine to TA Geneva Grey in Cheney Memorial. Rightmyer worked in this building on the night shift for the majority of her career as a nurse at Hudson River.

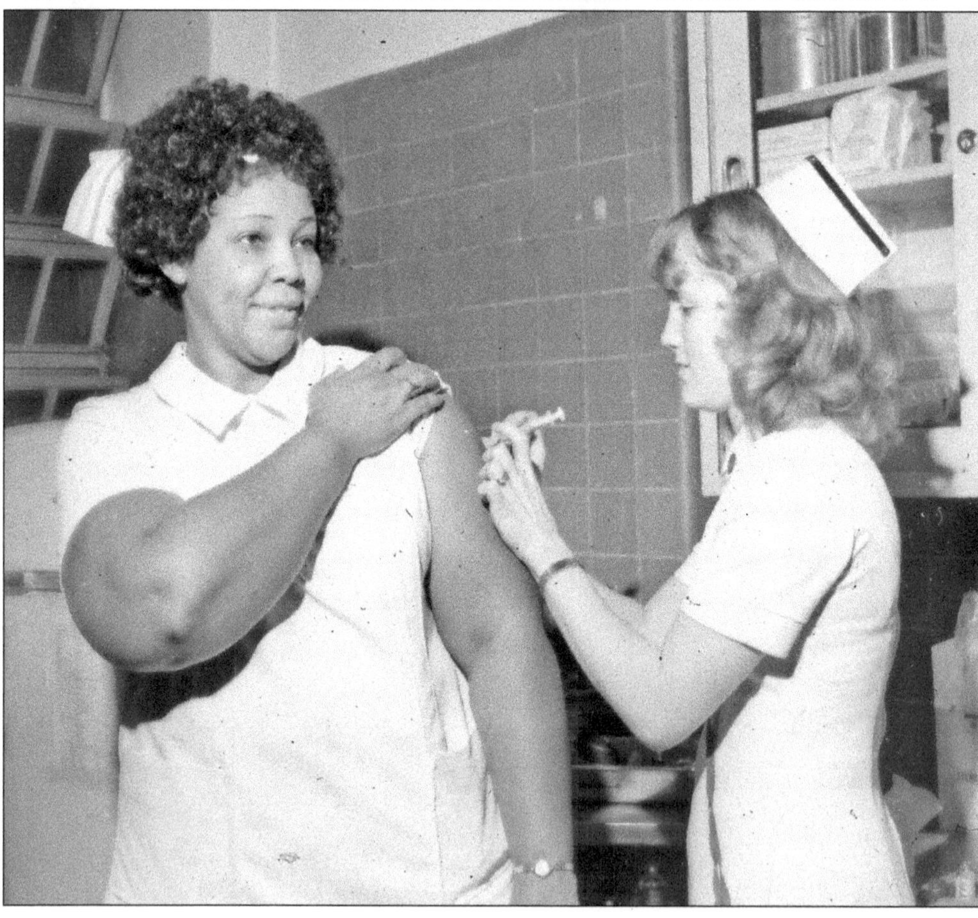

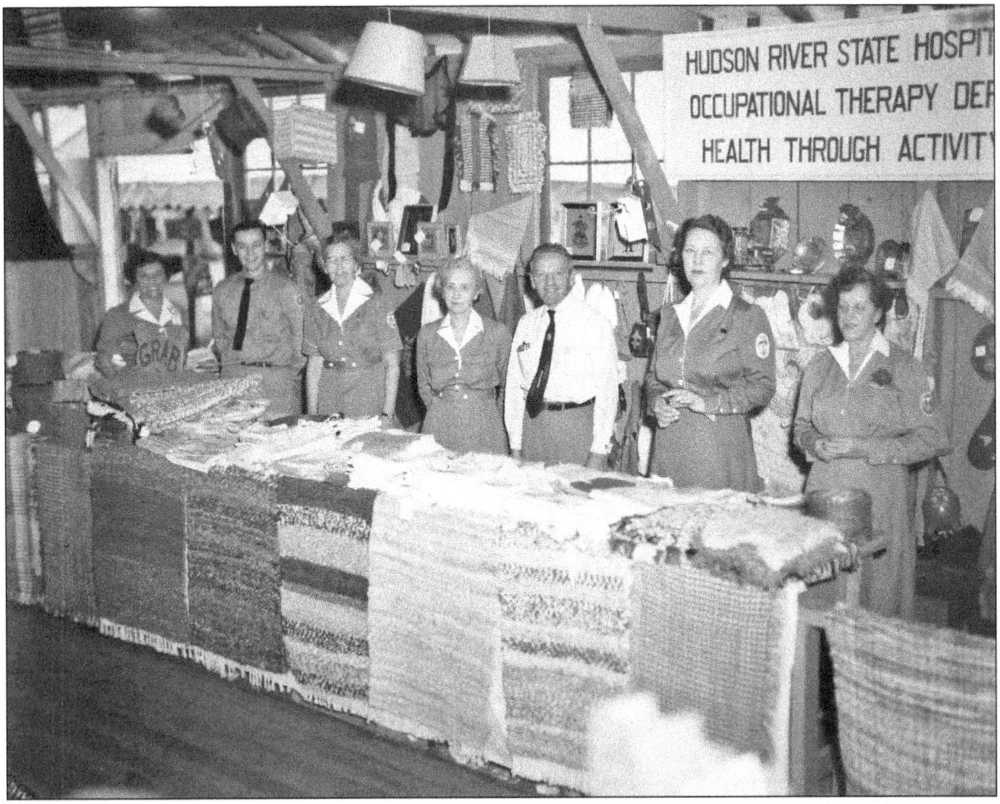

The hospital did not exist in a vacuum from the community surrounding it—in fact, that was the exact opposite intent of its creators. This 1957 photograph was taken at an occupational therapy exhibit at the Dutchess County Fair. Here the staff from the occupational therapy department proudly displays for sale many of the common articles made at Hudson River. Extra produce grown in August was brought for sale as well. Below, some of the prized crops farmers grew at Hudson River are on display. Canned and jarred products such as pickles were popular items produced at the hospital.

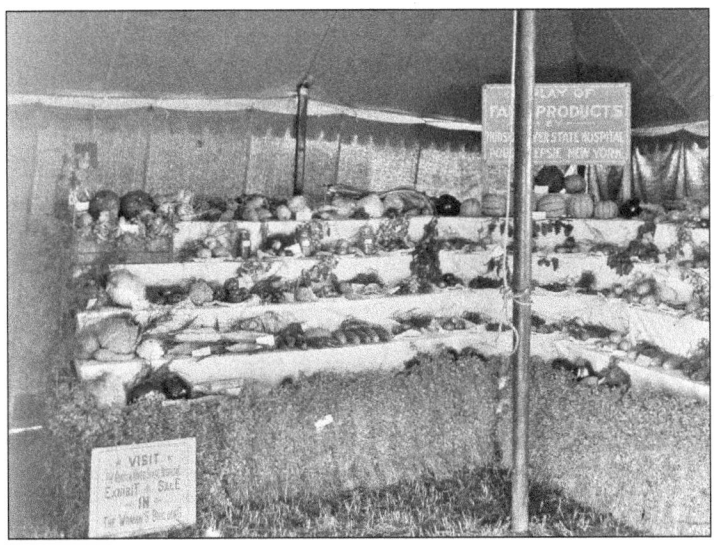

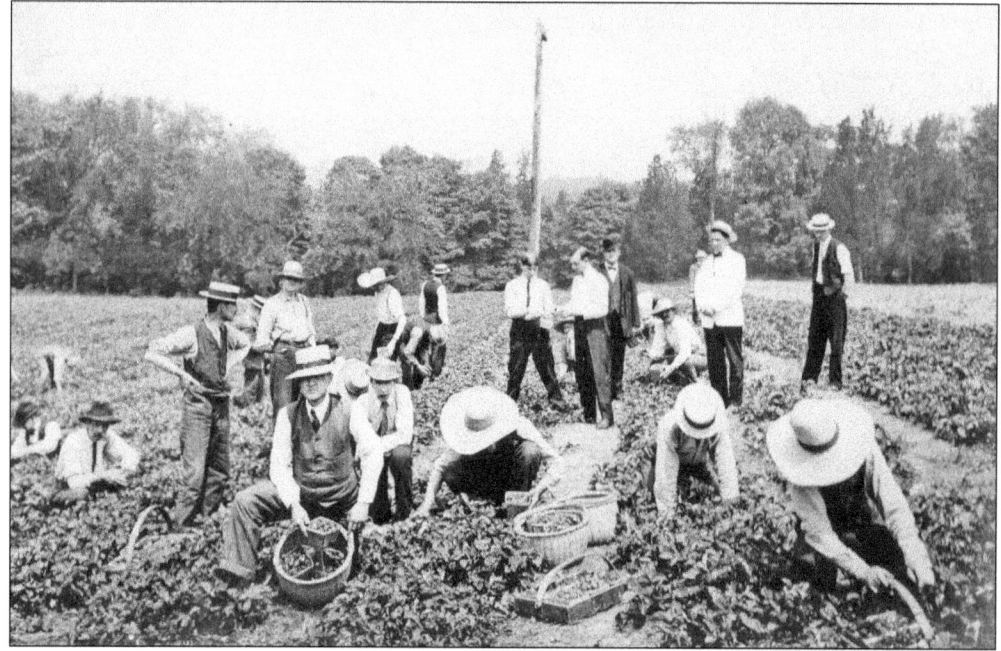

This spring photograph was taken in the 1920s at the hospital farm. Men are picking strawberries and putting them in pint containers. Even on a hot day performing labor, they wear collared shirts, ties, and vests. It is likely that not all of the people pictured are staff; some are probably patient workers assisting with the farm.

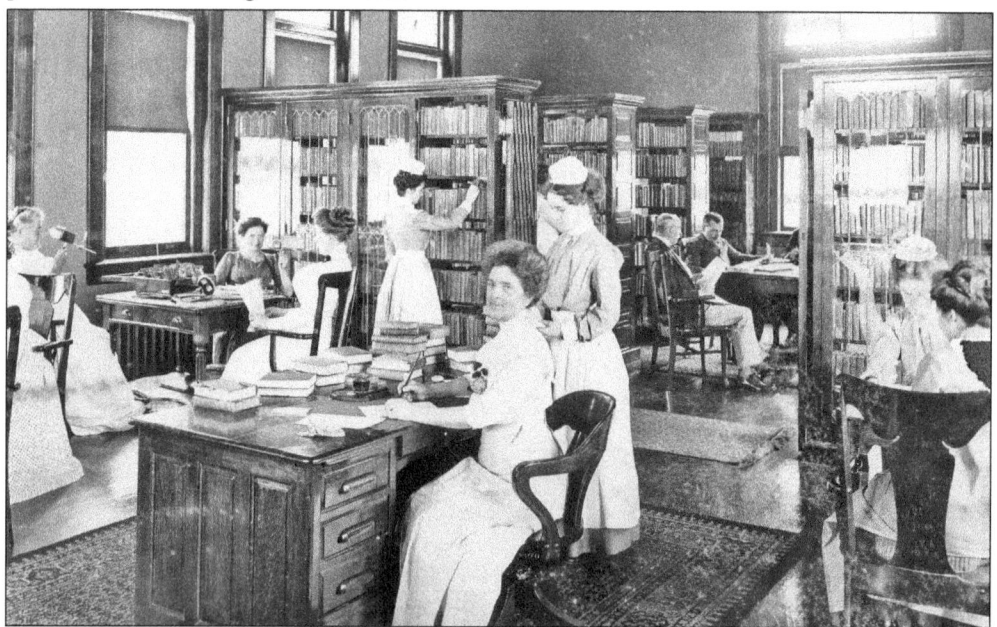

This photograph taken just after the turn of the century is of the staff library, which later became a patient library building. Up front at the desk facing the camera is the librarian, a Ms. Lounsberry. Even when not in formal work settings, men and women were expected to be dressed appropriately in hospital attire. This was one of few spaces at the time where men and women staff informally congregated during working hours.

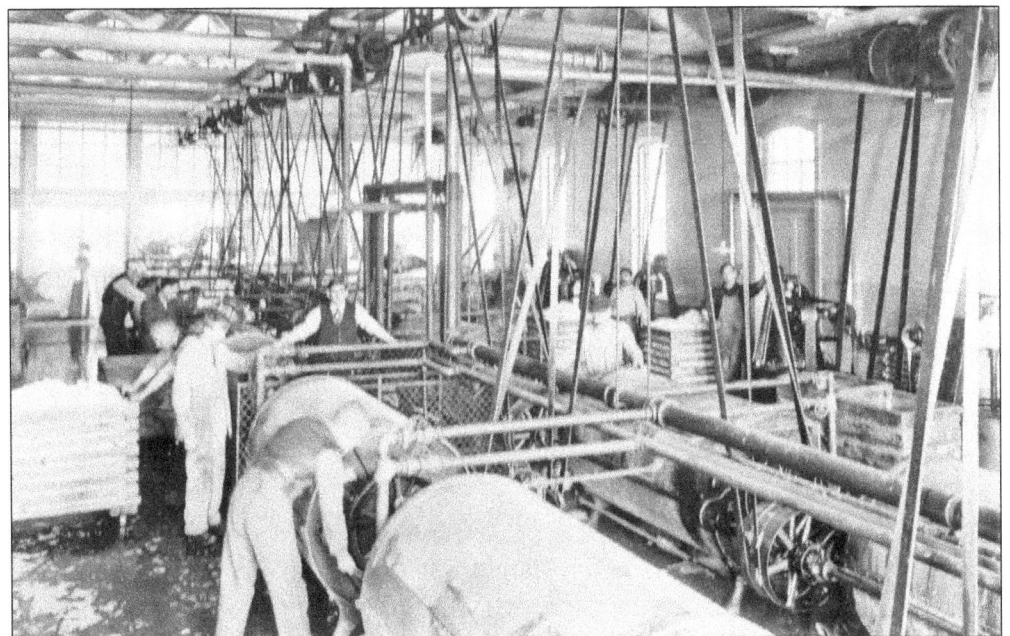

Even in laundry service, there was a segregation of males and females. This 1890s image shows the men's duties in the department. The large drums with belts attached are washing machines. Men did the heavier lifting of moving full carts of sorted clothing into washing and drying machines. At this time, the laundry was powered by steam turbines that turned the shaft spanning the length of the room.

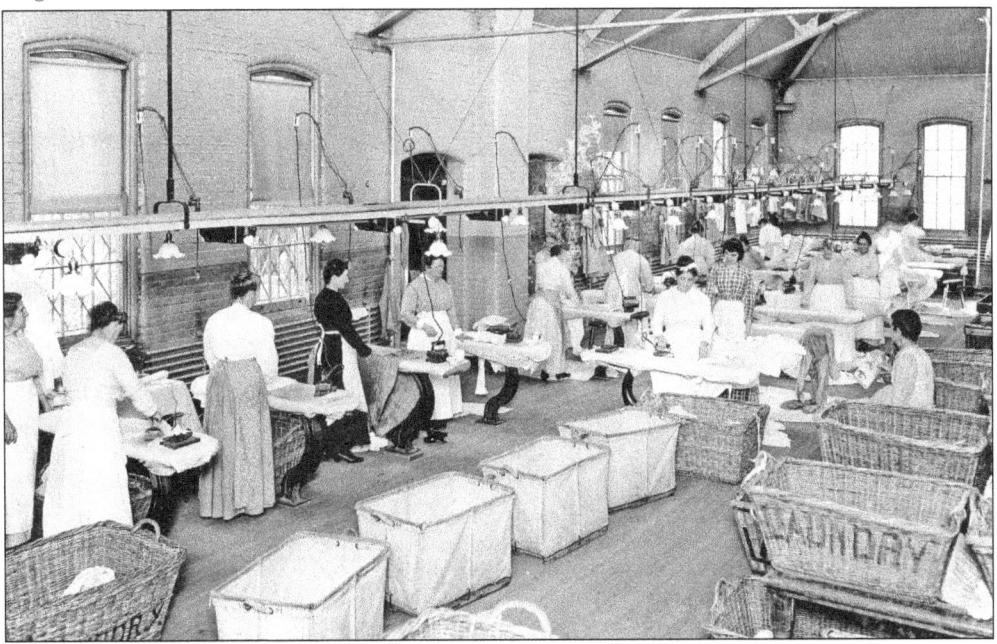

Women in laundry service also did hours of laborious work. All of the laundry was processed, separated, washed, and dried on site. This image shows female staff, likely aided by patient workers, ironing freshly washed laundry. Women were separated from men in this work detail. Sorting, folding, and ironing laundry were typical female work duties in this department.

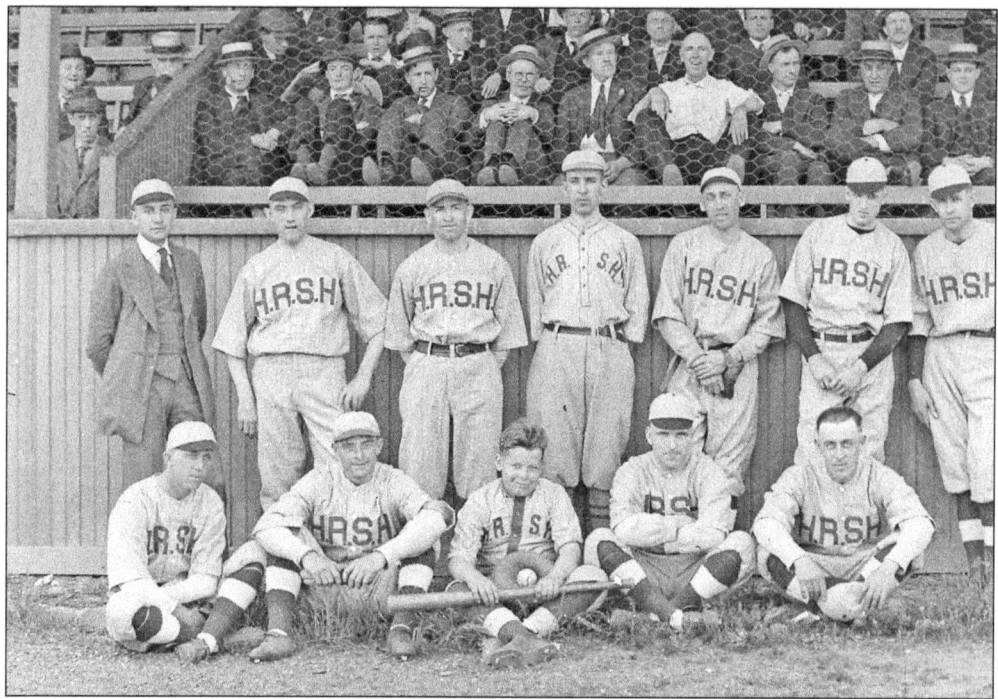

Baseball remained an American pastime long after the 1930s, when this photograph was taken. At the time, it certainly was the number-one sport of conversation and action in the country and at the state hospital. Leagues existed in state agencies for corrections, industries, and mental health, shown here. Different faculties in the same state department would compete for a title cup. Hudson River had its own grandstand, as many other facilities did, so staff and patients could watch practice and competitive games. Here, the men playing for Hudson River's ball team proudly stand shoulder to shoulder for a team photograph.

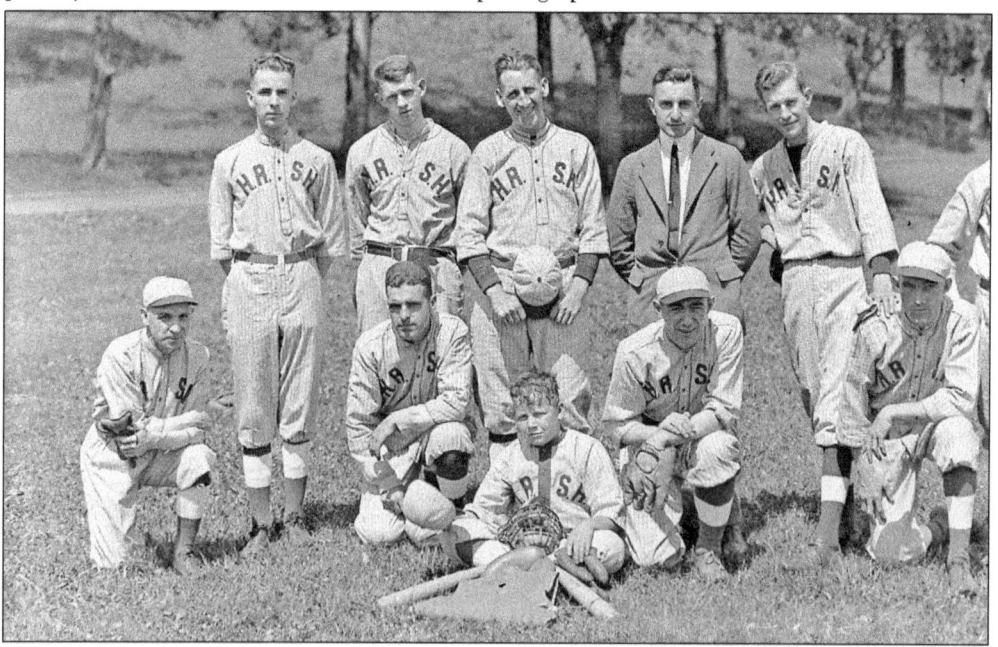

Here is one baseball trophy won in competition. This 1936 cup was a great source of pride for all the players, patients, and staff who cheered on their home team. Not only was this a fun activity for all, it was a way of uniting staff and patients over common ground. Social activities like this were part of creating a community of care in the hospital.

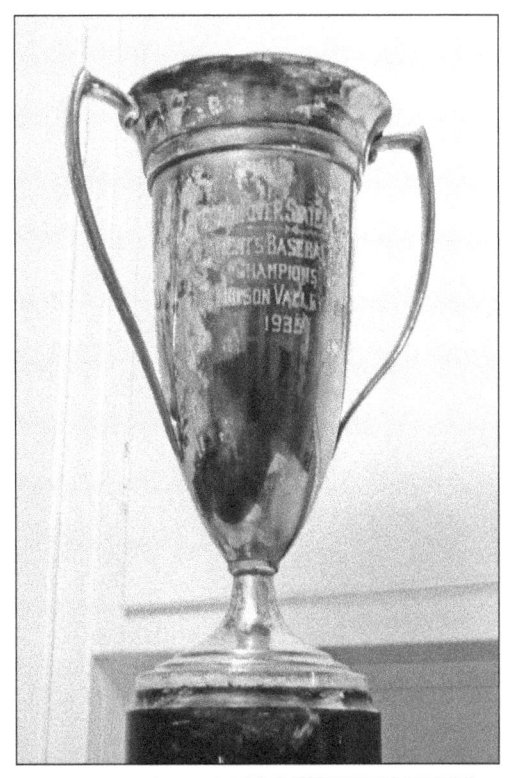

A board of visitors was established a few years after opening Hudson River. This was a body of local volunteer dignitaries who would inspect the hospital for proper conditions. They had their own keys and made rounds unannounced. James Roosevelt, father of Pres. Franklin Roosevelt, served on the board for several years. In the 1890s, this board of visitors poses for a photograph.

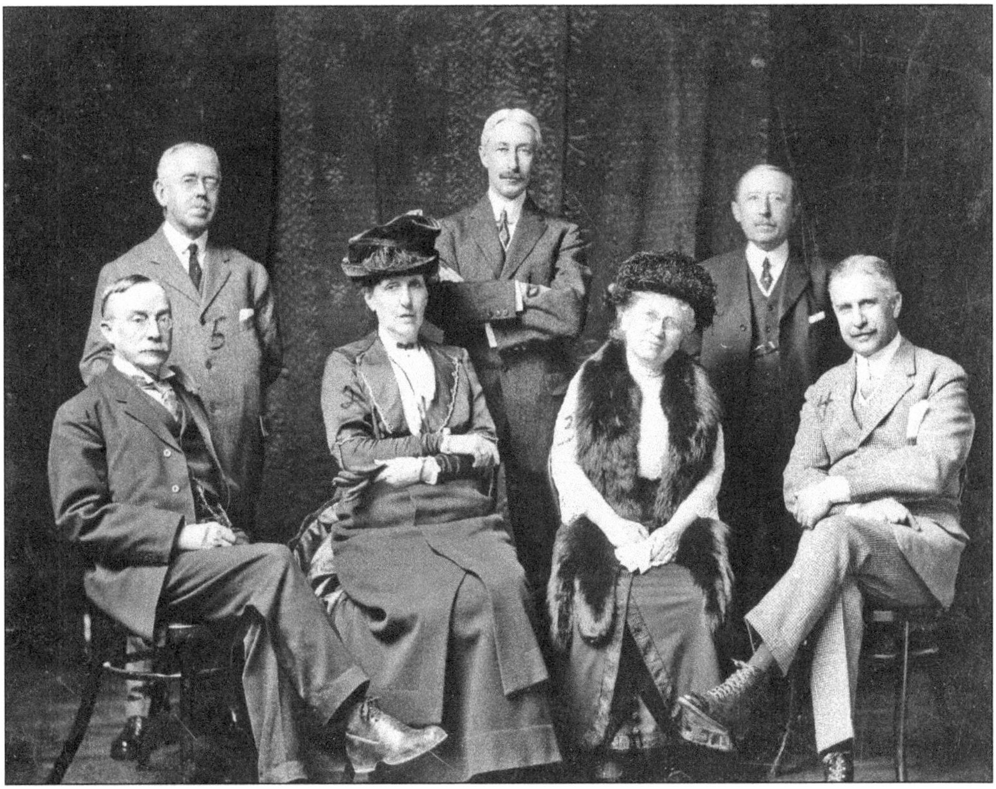

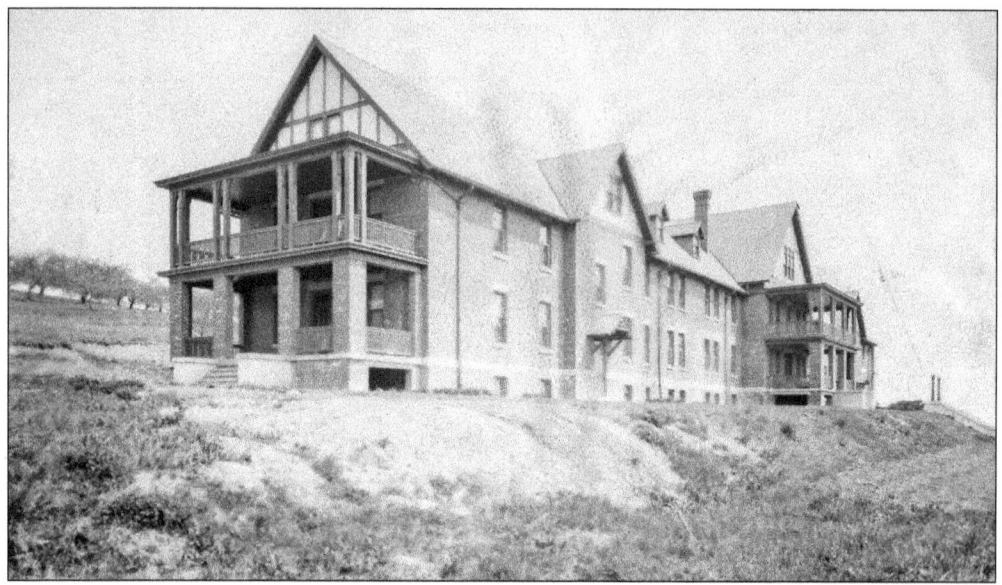

Named for the hospital's first superintendent, Joseph M. Cleveland, this building was erected in 1924 as apartments for single staff. Mostly attendants lived here in a dorm setting. Rooms were small and had enough space for a bed, dresser, small table, and a sink with a mirror. Toilets and showers were shared by the floor, along with a common area for socializing.

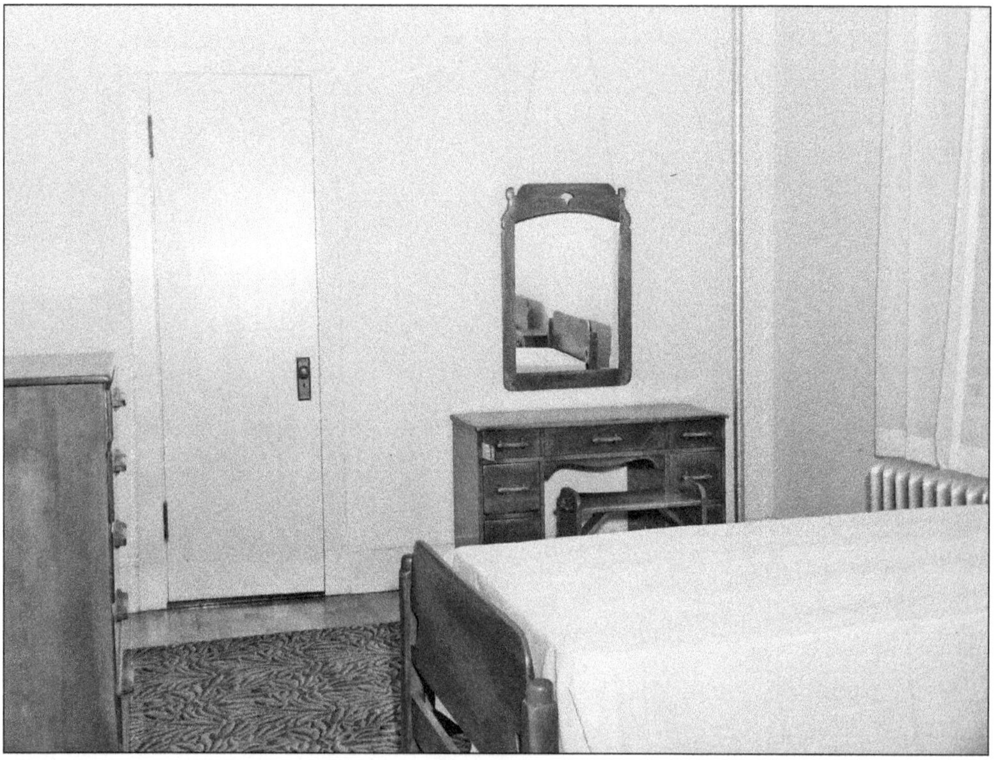

Shown in October 1951 is an apartment at the northern end of Cleveland Home. This was single attendant housing. Here a newly furnished living room space is shown. Two staff of the same sex would have roomed here and shared this common area.

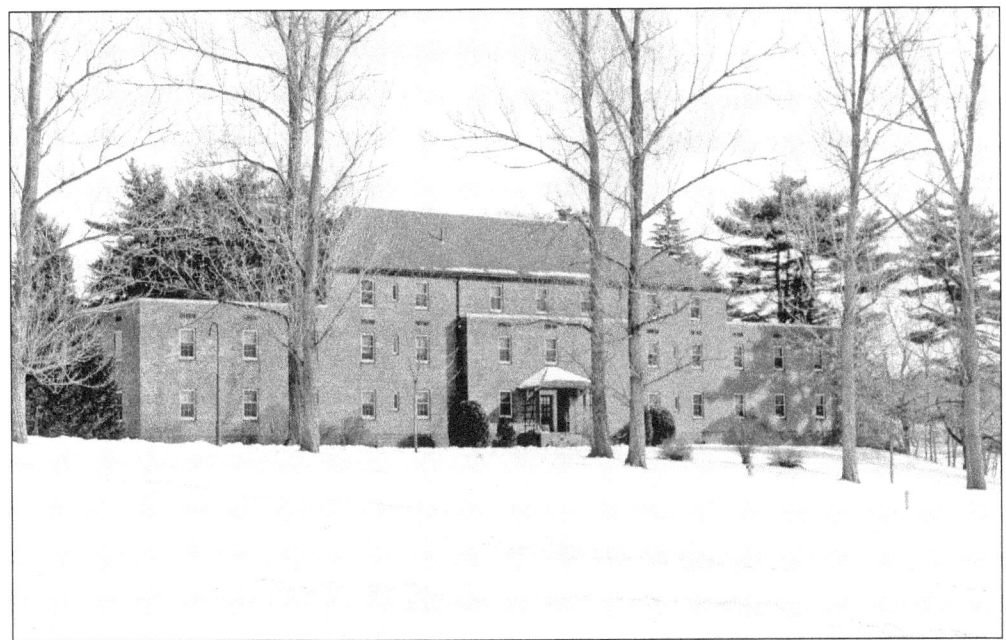

Avery Home opened in 1931 to house staff. This was a home for student nurses. Rooms were generally shared by two students as one would find in a college dormitory. Each student nurse home had a house mother, who would act as a resident attendant, enforcing rules and keeping order. Student nurses had a curfew and were forbidden from having men in their rooms.

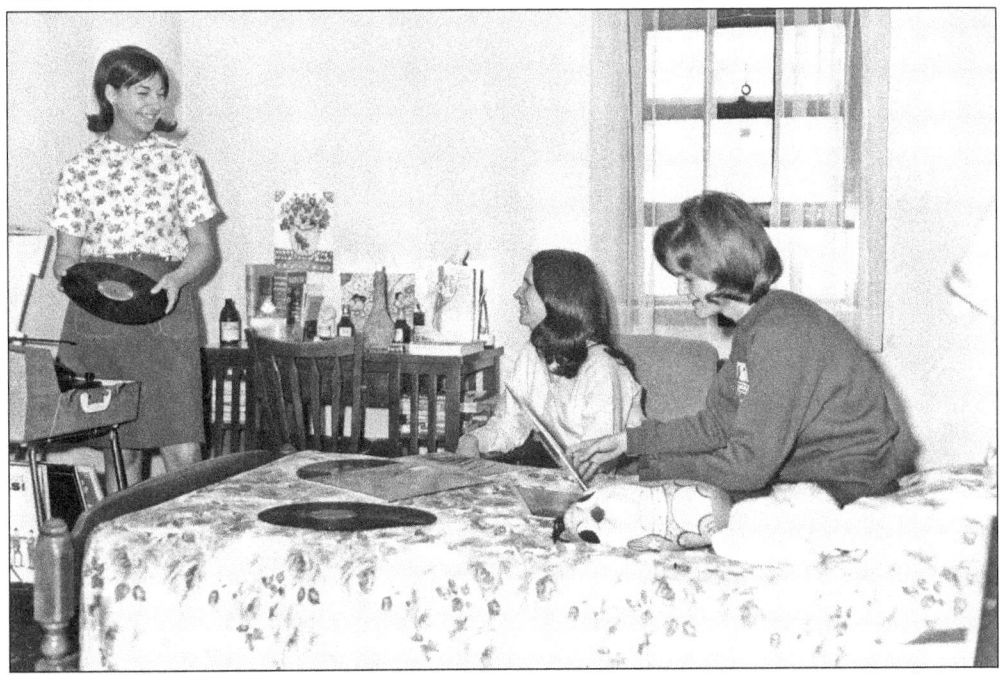

These smiling young ladies at Hudson River are student nurses. The nursing school was an attractive program that drew youth from all over the state. Room and board were offered on top of education and a guaranteed job at the hospital. Here, in what appears to be Avery Home, one young lady selects a record to play.

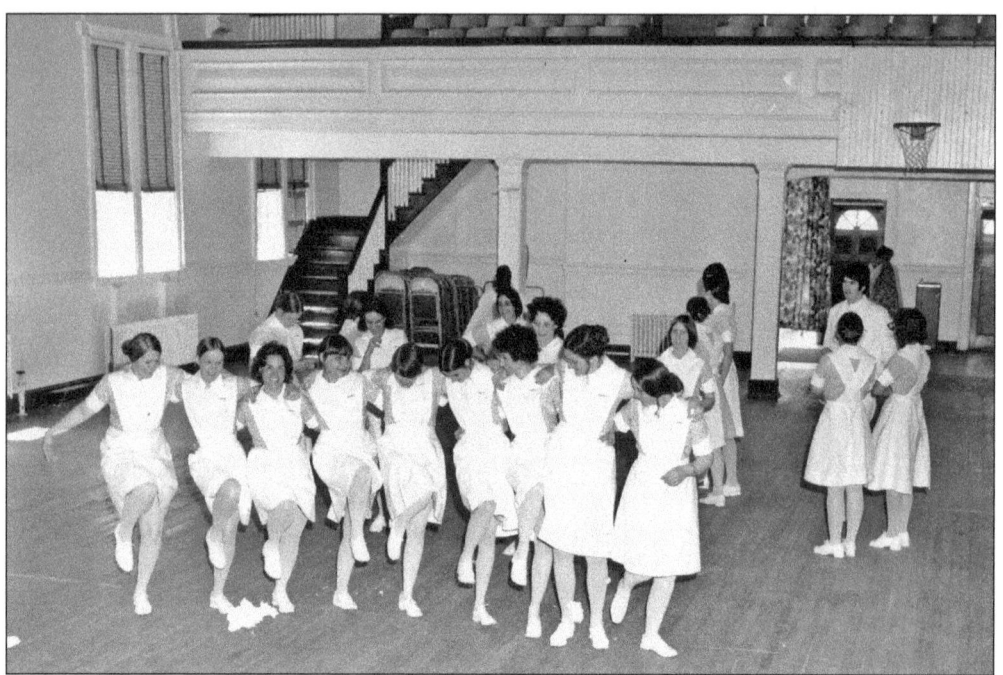

Quartering and working at the hospital in the 1950s was more than a job, it was a social way of life. The nursing school was a similar experience to what young men and women would find at a college but with more discipline. Recreation and laughter was the chief prescription of the day for a long and stressful workday. Here a group of student nurses dances about the Assembly Hall.

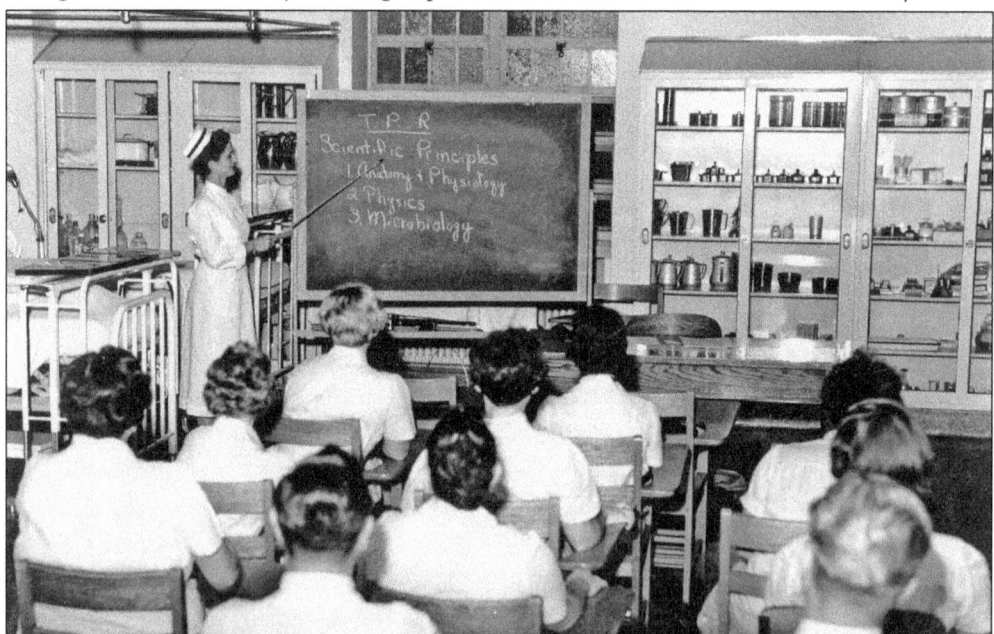

Continuing education and training were a part of life for all staff. Annual classes were held for ward personnel to stay current in medical or psychiatric treatment practices. In this photograph in Cheney Memorial, student nurses are being instructed by a nurse on temperature, pulse, and respiration measurement.

Three
NURSING AND TREATMENT

When the hospital received its first patient in 1871, the principle treatment was moral therapy. This centered around a stimulating environment, vocation, art, music, and congregate activity. Early medications used were paraldehyde, bromide, chloral, and luminal along with various tonics. Effectiveness was not extraordinary, as these agents did not act on receptors in the brain associated with psychosis. Hydrotherapy was common for disturbed patients to induce a calming effect. Contrary to common beliefs, many patients were discharged prior to the advent of psychiatric medication in 1955. Common sense dictates that being removed from the stressful environment that triggered an emotional illness would be beneficial to recovery. Nevertheless, research and work to provide best treatment practices has been a focus of Hudson River State Hospital since its inception.

Nursing service provided the backbone of the hospital. Attendants and nurse staff made up the largest number of hospital personnel by far. Logistically, this made sense, as the nursing department was responsible for staffing the facility 24 hours a day. On August 31, 1886, the hospital established its own nurse training school under Dr. Cleveland. This program was to train nurses specifically in care and treatment of the "insane." The nursing school officially closed its doors in 1977, graduating its final class on December 5 that year. During the 91 years of operation at Hudson River, the training school graduated 229 men and 833 women. In the early days of the program, women were paid $10 to $17 per month and men $16 to $22 per month. Students received a comprehensive education as they rotated through general hospitals to receive specialized training in obstetrics, pediatrics, surgery, and contagious diseases.

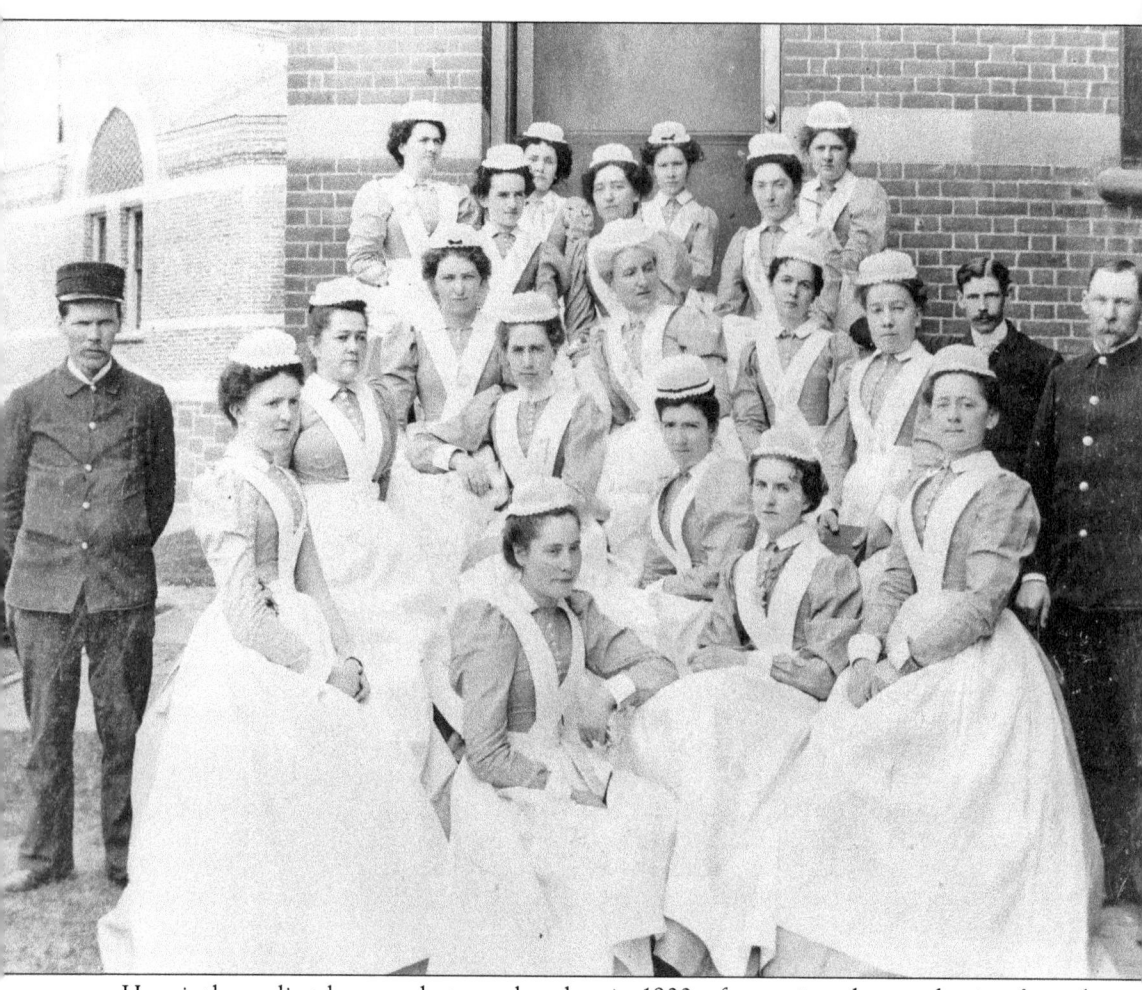

Here is the earliest known photograph, taken in 1900, of a nursing class graduating from the nursing training school at Hudson River State Hospital. The exterior of the main building makes up the background. The nursing school remained here until newer buildings were constructed in the 20th century. This class still wears the same uniform as when the hospital began the training school in 1886. Men, as graduation numbers reflect, were generally outnumbered by women in this profession at Hudson River. For women, a uniform of a blue dress with a white bib and cap was protocol. As the years went on at Hudson River, the uniform changed a number of times. By the 1980s, staff for the most part no longer wore uniforms but plain street clothes.

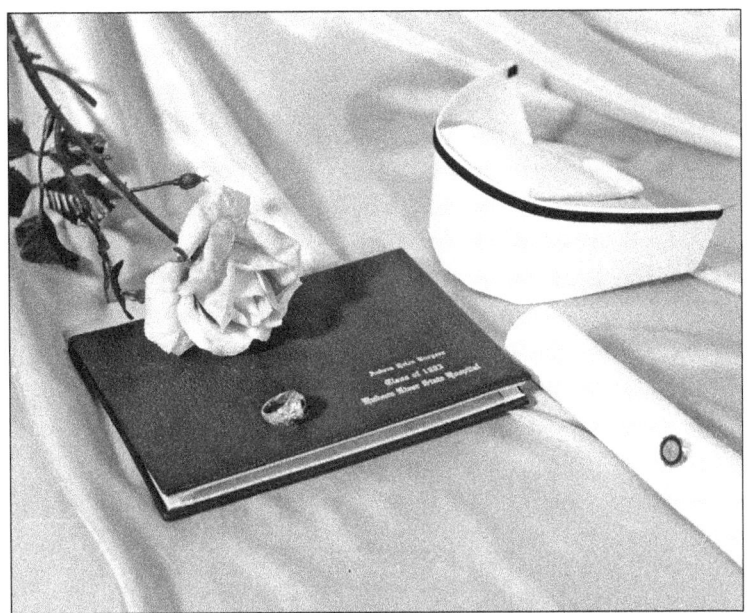

This 1960s photograph shows the items a recipient of the school of nursing was presented with upon commencement. The graduated nurse's cap had one black stripe. While working on the wards as a student nurse, the cap had two blue stripes with a gold stripe in the middle. Pins commonly were affixed to the nurse's cape lapel.

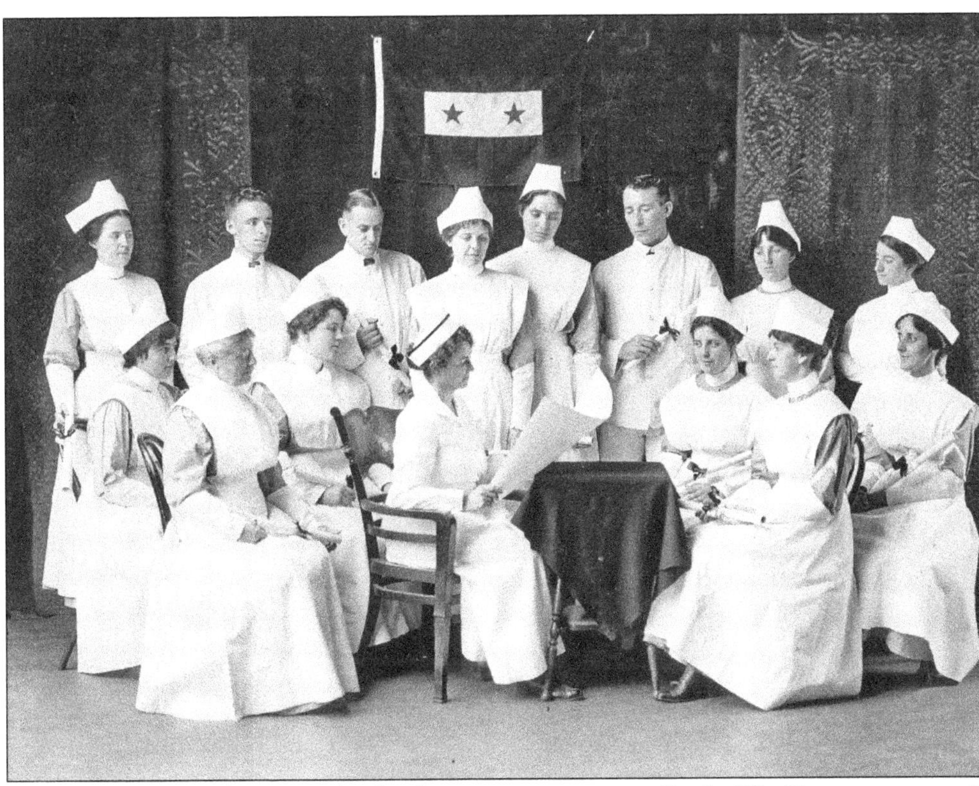

In an effort to aid soldiers injured in battle, nurses were recruited by the War Department to assist in World War I. In the background of this photograph of the class of 1918, two blue stars hang on a flag representing nurses from Hudson River who were abroad assisting the war effort.

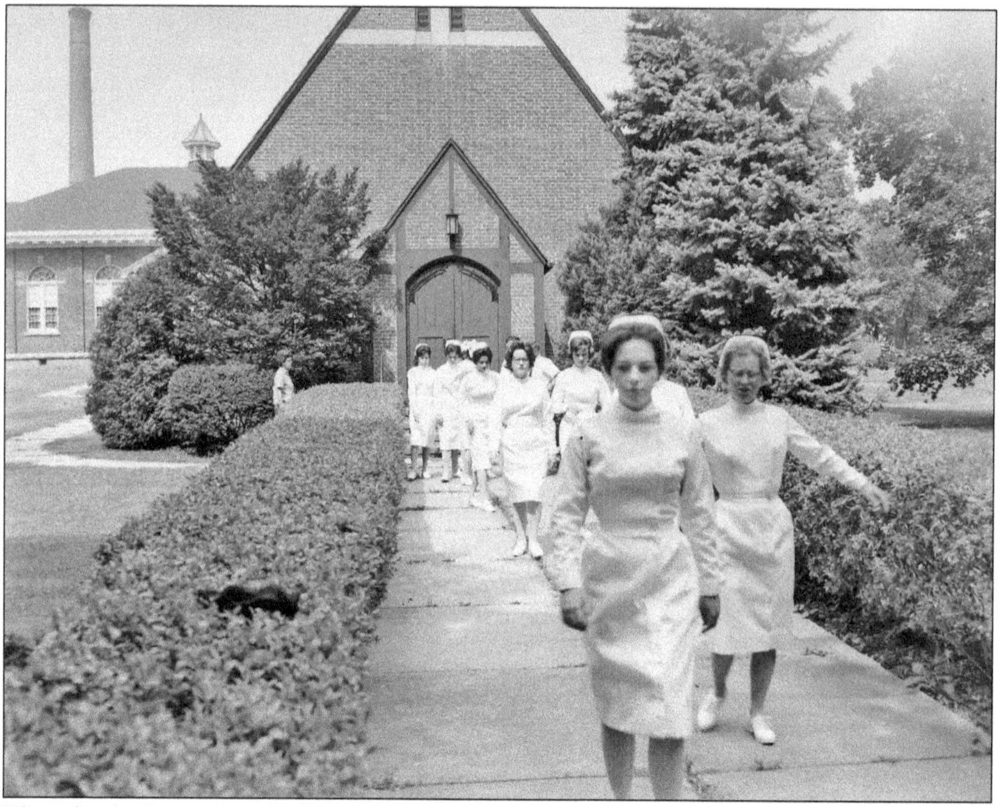

The school of nursing at Hudson River was held to the same standards as any other accredited nursing program at the time. In the early years, graduates received certificates that allowed them to work in any other state hospital in New York. In later years, local colleges offered certificate to degree programs, allowing registered nurses to attain an accredited degree. This photograph shows the recently graduated class of 1963 at Hudson River, including Linda Hacksteiner (third from rear on the left), today a retired nurse administrator, active corresponding secretary, and curator with the Hudson River State Hospital Nurses Alumni Association. Also identified are Margaret Littlefield and Janile Ek-Grubs (left and right to the right of Hacksteiner).

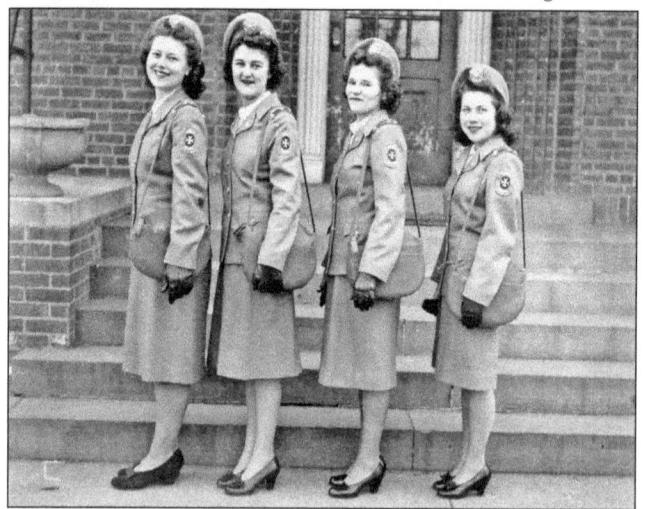

As in World War I, World War II brought forward a need for nurses in the battlefield and military hospitals. The cadet corps of nurses at Hudson River left hospital service to aid the war effort at home and abroad. Here the military-bound women of the hospital are ready to embark during World War II.

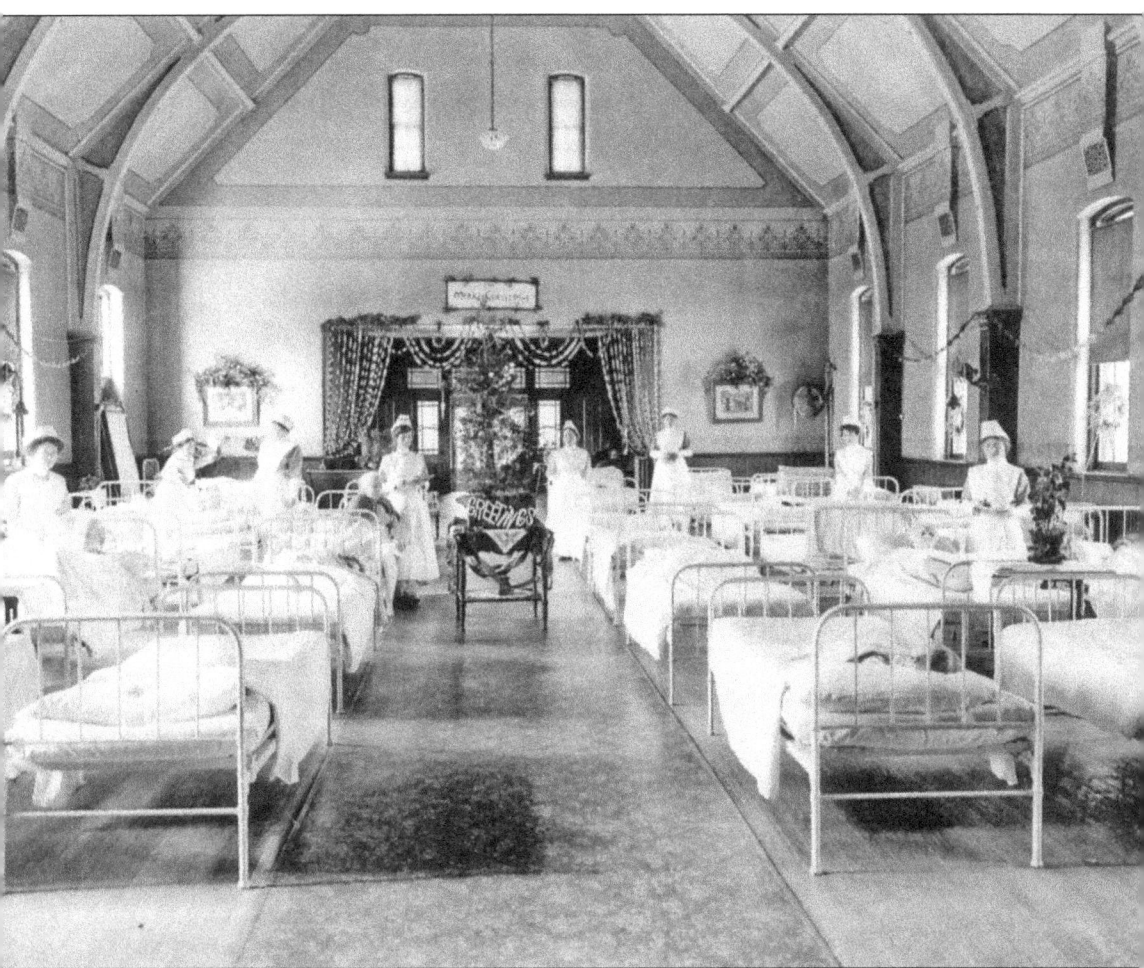

Sections of the main building changed purposes several times over the years. This early-1900s photograph taken in the north wing shows a ward for infirm women. It was a matter of considerable importance to adorn wards in cheerful decorations for the holidays, especially Christmas. Since most of the patients on this type of unit were bedridden, large day hall spaces were not incorporated into the design. This had been the Assembly Hall for the hospital until a separate building was constructed behind the main building. As time went on and more buildings were erected, this space would ultimately become a storage area for the maintenance department. If one looks closely at the walls, the decorative paint and molding from the room's previous use can be identified. The high ceilings with decorative iron beams certainly made it an ornate room for living quarters.

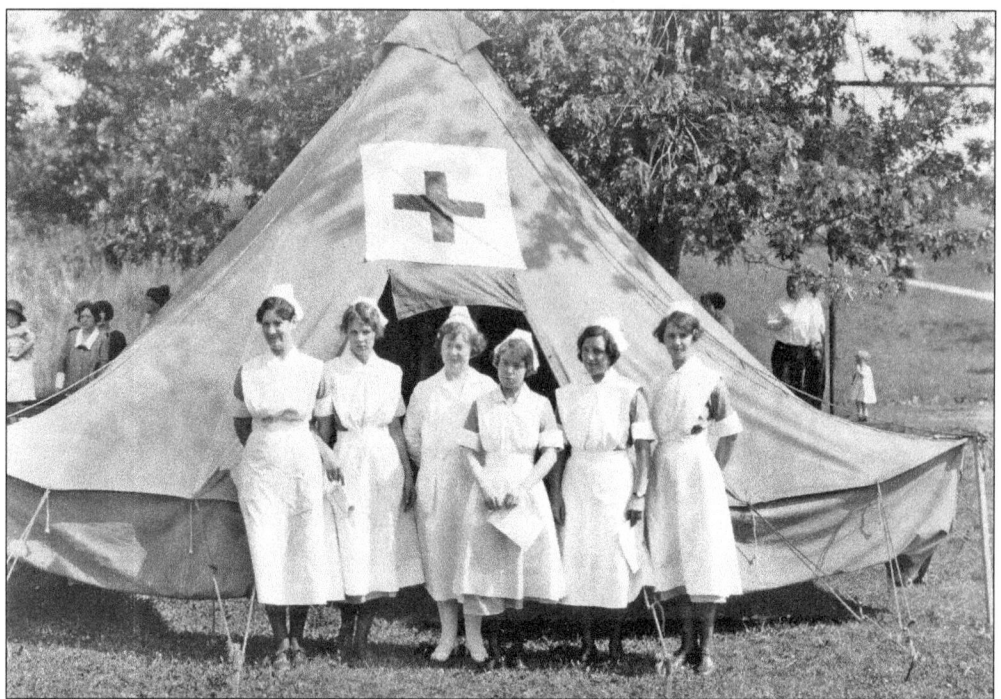

Disaster drills were commonplace from elementary schools to hospitals for many decades. Emergency management plans were drafted all over the state and simulated through drill. This 1927 photograph shows a mock disaster relief tent set up during field day exercises at Hudson River.

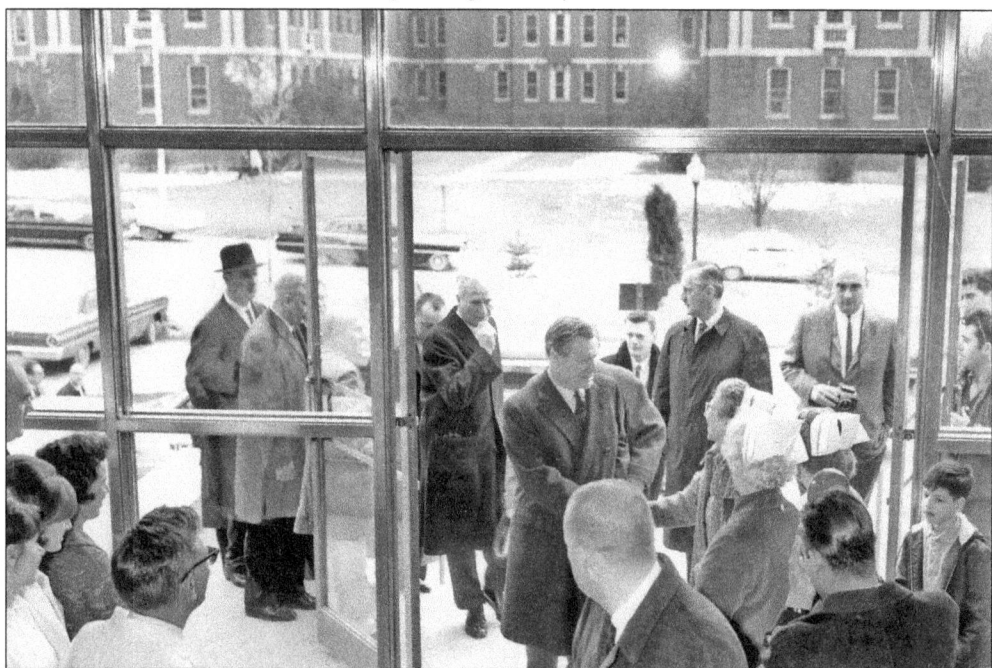

This 1960s image could be found in the state newsletters of the day. Governor Rockefeller was photographed as he entered the lobby of Cheney Memorial to tour the wards of the hospital. Most of his time that day was spent with the nursing department staff or in areas that nursing oversaw.

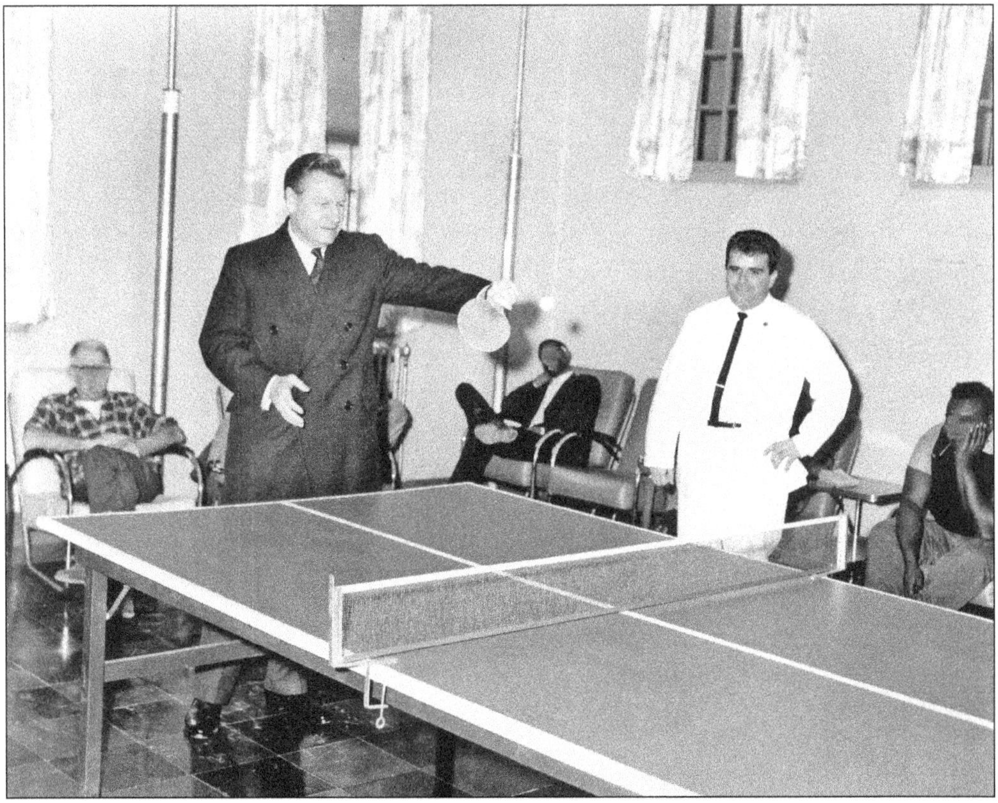

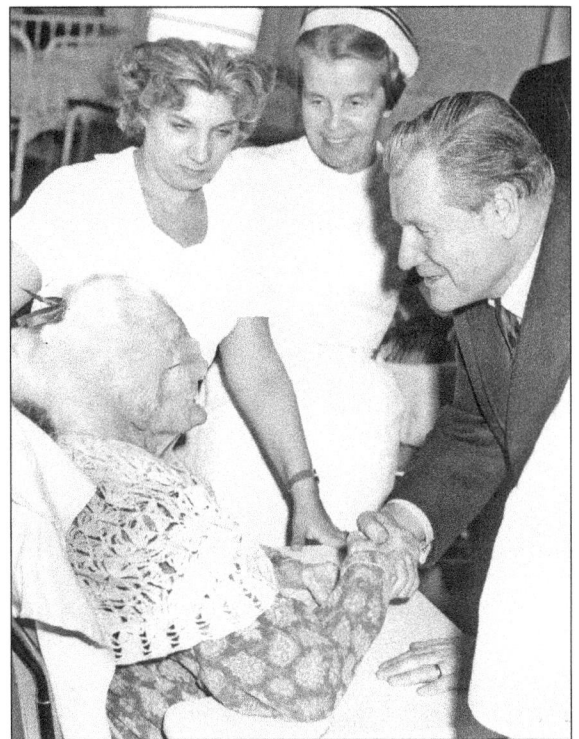

These two photographs were taken on the same day when the governor visited Hudson River. Above, Governor Rockefeller challenges patients to a game of Ping-Pong he vigorously engages in. In conversation with several individuals who worked with the governor personally, he was described as "genuine." This author suspects that, cameras following Governor Rockefeller or not that day, he would have behaved exactly the same. At right, Governor Rockefeller shakes the hand of a 100-year-old female patient on her birthday. This was undoubtedly a very happy moment for this woman, as many patients did not have family who visited.

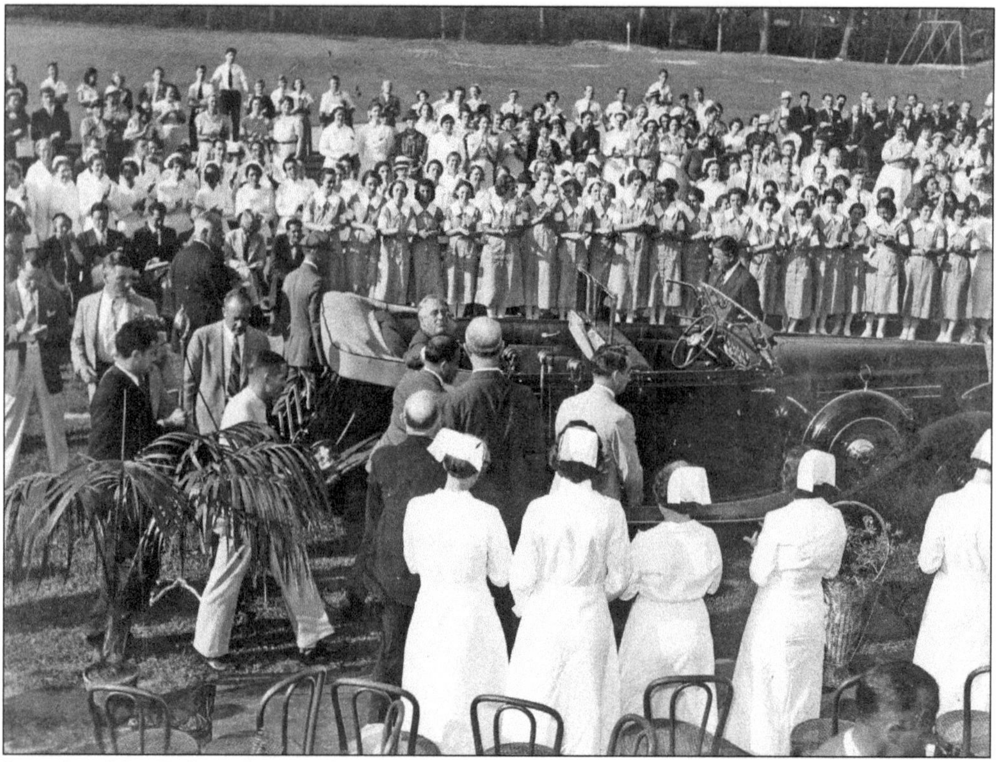

Pres. Franklin Delano Roosevelt was no stranger to Hudson River. His father, James, was the proprietor of the land the hospital was built upon and served on the board of managers for more than 20 years beginning in 1873. In a speech while president of the United States, he described his trips to Hudson River with his father, where FDR would "hold the horses" for James Roosevelt as he went into ward buildings. Above, FDR visits in 1935 to speak at the commencement ceremonies for a nursing school graduation. Below, President Roosevelt can be seen delivering a keynote at the commencement ceremony.

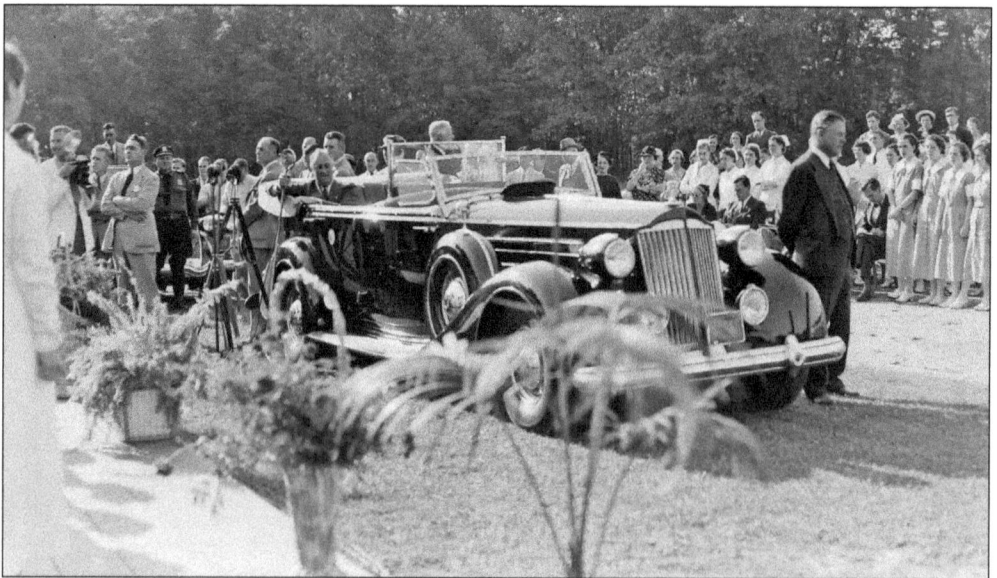

Even after living many miles away from their family home in Hyde Park year-round in New York City, the Roosevelts kept in contact with Hudson River. Former first lady Eleanor Roosevelt also spoke at nursing school graduations. This was a great source of local pride for the hospital and often attracted positive media attention. This 1960 letter from Eleanor Roosevelt informs of her intent to provide a keynote speech for a September graduation that year; interestingly enough, she requested more information be sent about the history of the facility and nursing school.

MRS. FRANKLIN D. ROOSEVELT
55 EAST 74TH STREET
NEW YORK CITY 21, N. Y.

RECEIVED
AUG 23 1960
HUDSON RIVER STA

August 20, 1960

Dear Dr. Hunt:

I look forward to being with you on September 16th and I hope you will send me some historical background material. Please note on the material that it is for September 16th as my secretary and I are leaving for a trip abroad and will not return until September 14th when a welter of material will greet us.

I do not need transportation.

With many thanks and my good wishes,

Very sincerely yours,

Eleanor Roosevelt

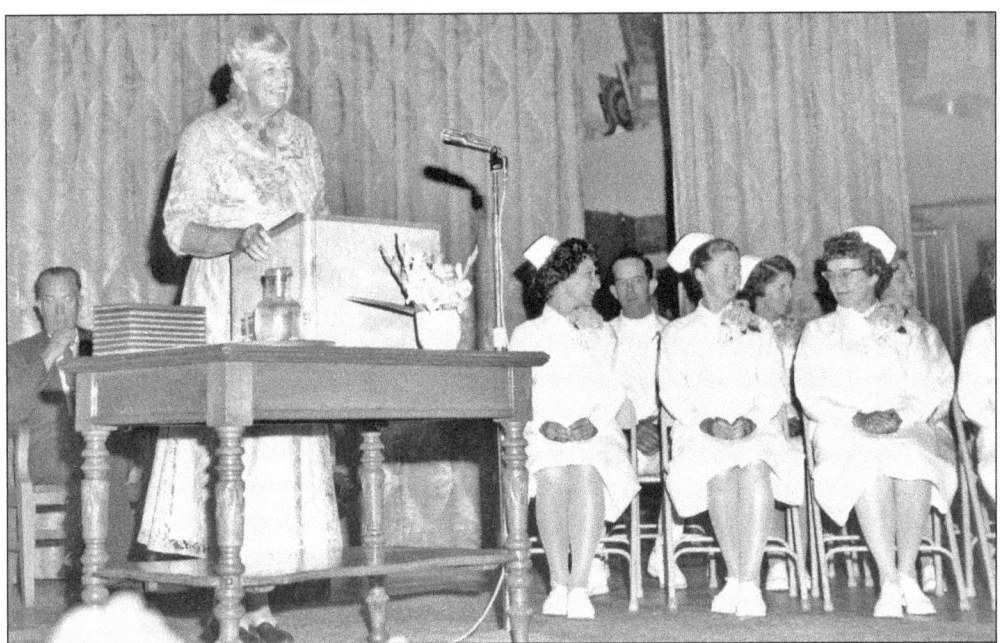

Eleanor Roosevelt is shown speaking at that September 1960 graduation. To the right, a group of excited student nurses listens to the speech.

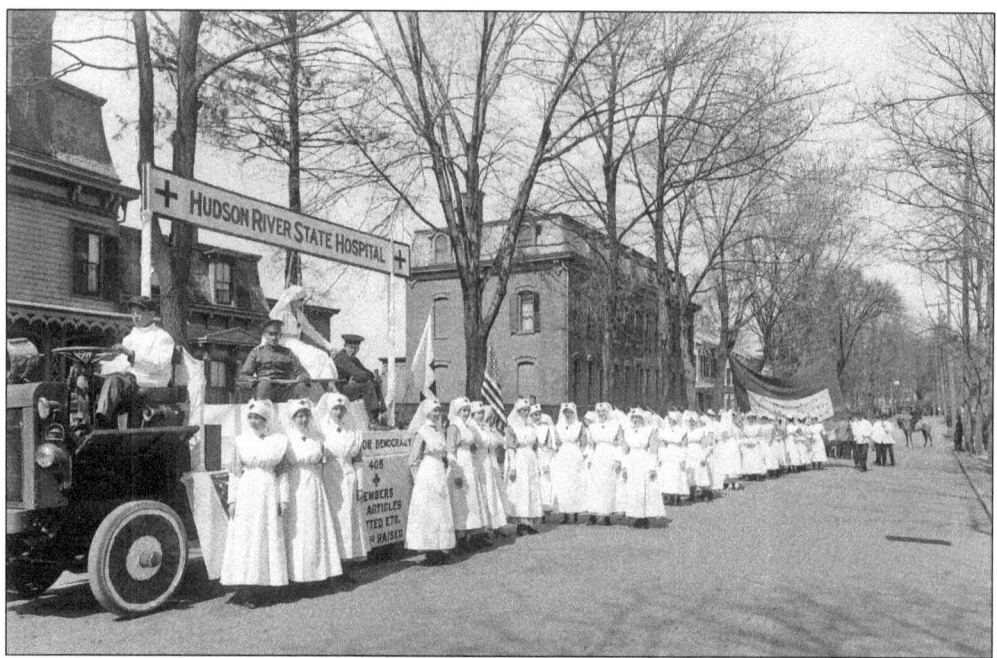

During the life of Hudson River State Hospital, it is fair to say that there was a level of pride taken in the hospital, evidenced by the physical condition and standards of treatment. Nursing service stands out in terms of loudly voicing their satisfaction in the facility not only as an employer but also often as their alma mater. In this 1918 Liberty Day parade in Poughkeepsie, the nursing staff proudly displays their role in psychiatric care. During World War I, this parade was not only to showcase hospital pride but also displayed its proud American identity. The tank float displays the value of Liberty Bonds sold at Hudson River State Hospital to support the war effort.

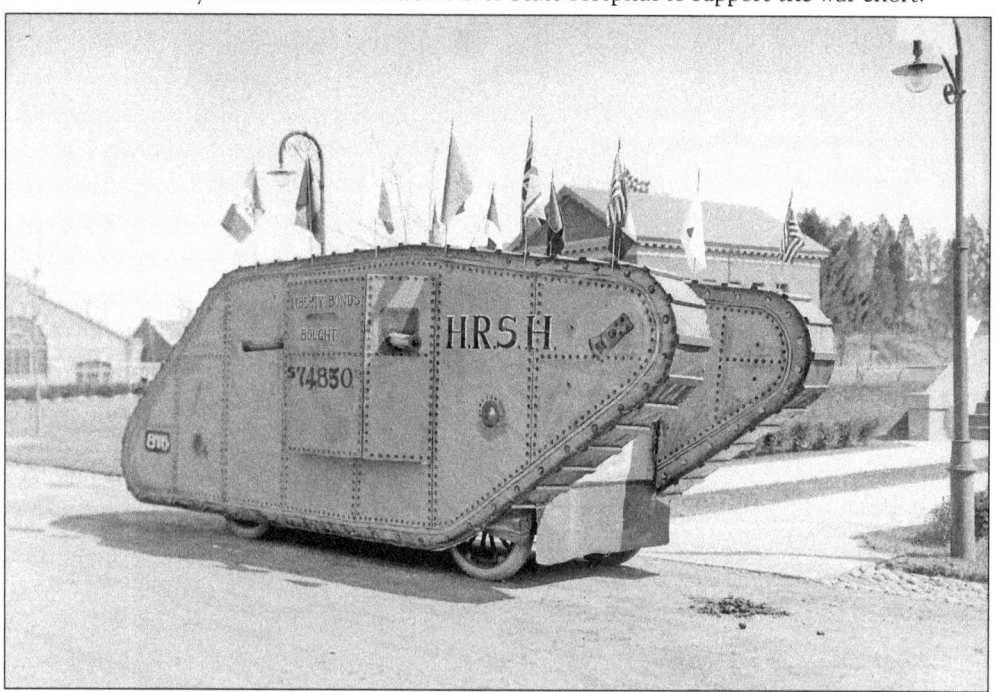

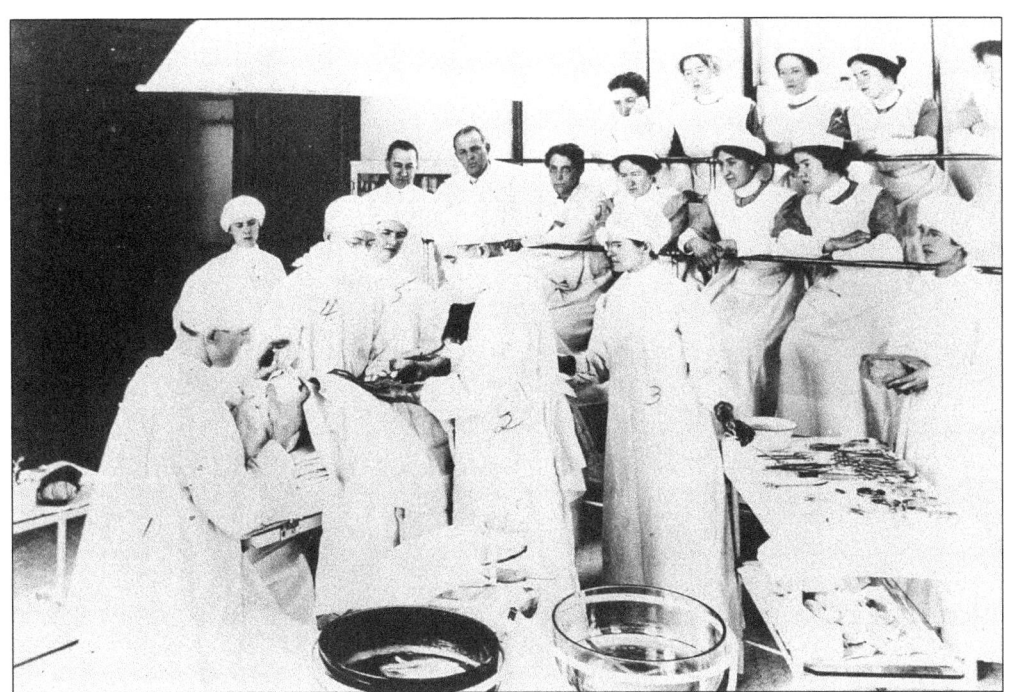

As part of a comprehensive training program, nurses attended open surgeries. A select few were assigned to work in the medical and surgical services at Hudson River. The above photograph, taken around the turn of the century, shows an operation in the main building. Although some nurses would go on to specialize in operative care, it was imperative for all those working in this profession to have a working understanding of surgery and aftercare. The 1960s photograph below shows a doctor with two operating room nurses at one of Cheney Memorial's operating suites. After the construction of the operating services in Cheney, all other surgical suites on the property were decommissioned.

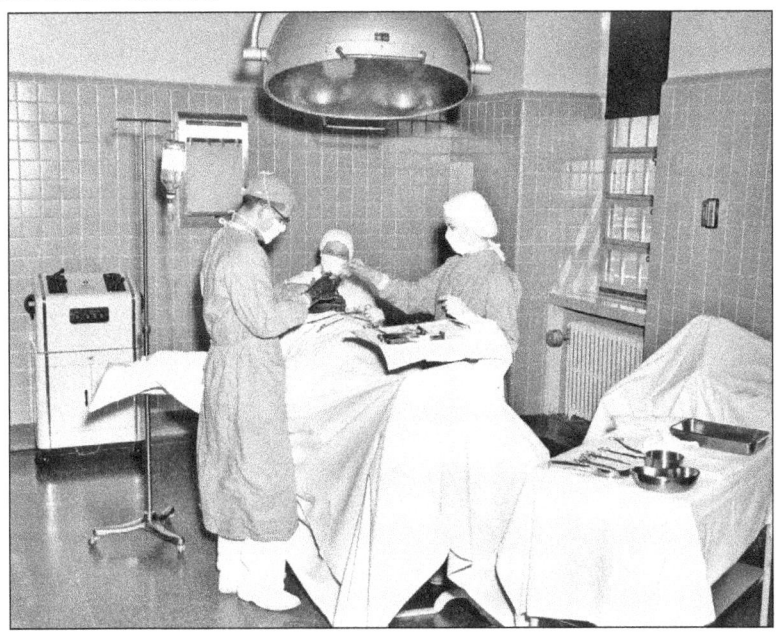

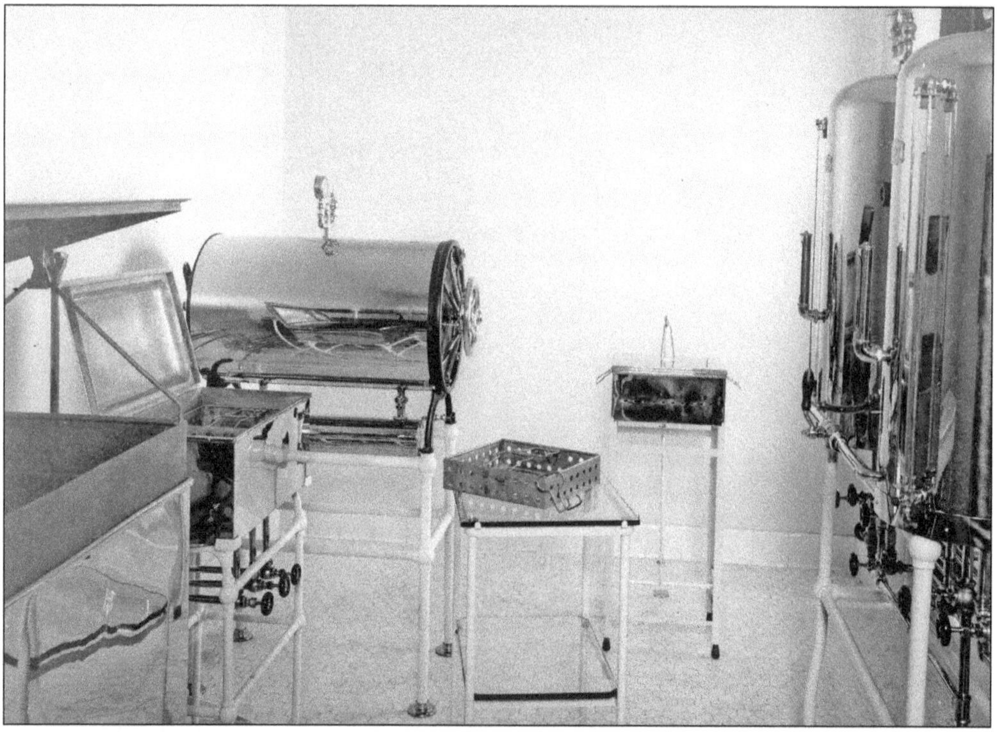

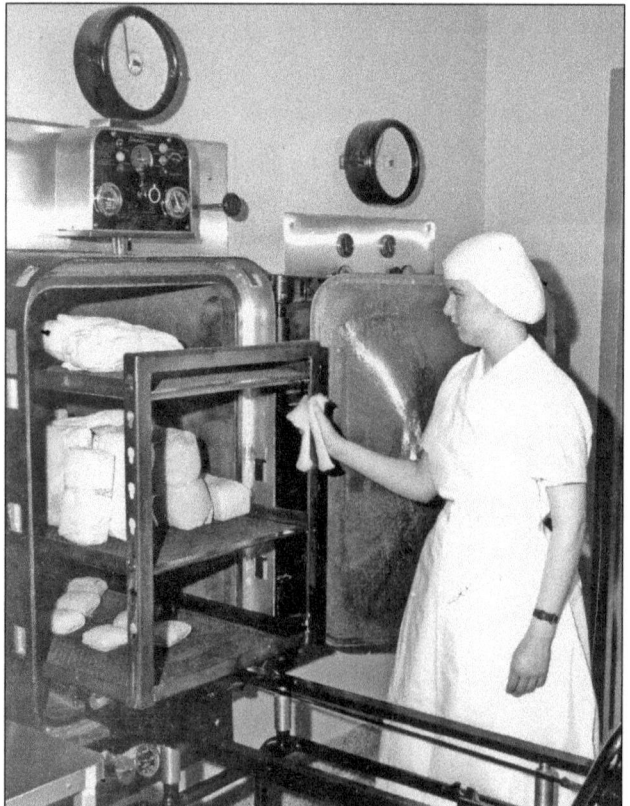

This 1912 image was taken in the main building adjacent to the operating suite. After the operating room was removed from this building, the business office occupied this renovated location. Here, new state-of-the-art sterilizing equipment is proudly displayed. This photograph was taken for an early publication at the hospital describing equipment and techniques in medical instrument cleaning.

To prevent the spread of disease and ensure general cleanliness of medical instruments, sterilization was done in house with an autoclave, essentially a steam-powered, pressurized unit that kills any living microbes. Here in Cheney Memorial in the 1960s, a staff member can be seen removing medical instruments wrapped in towels after sterilization.

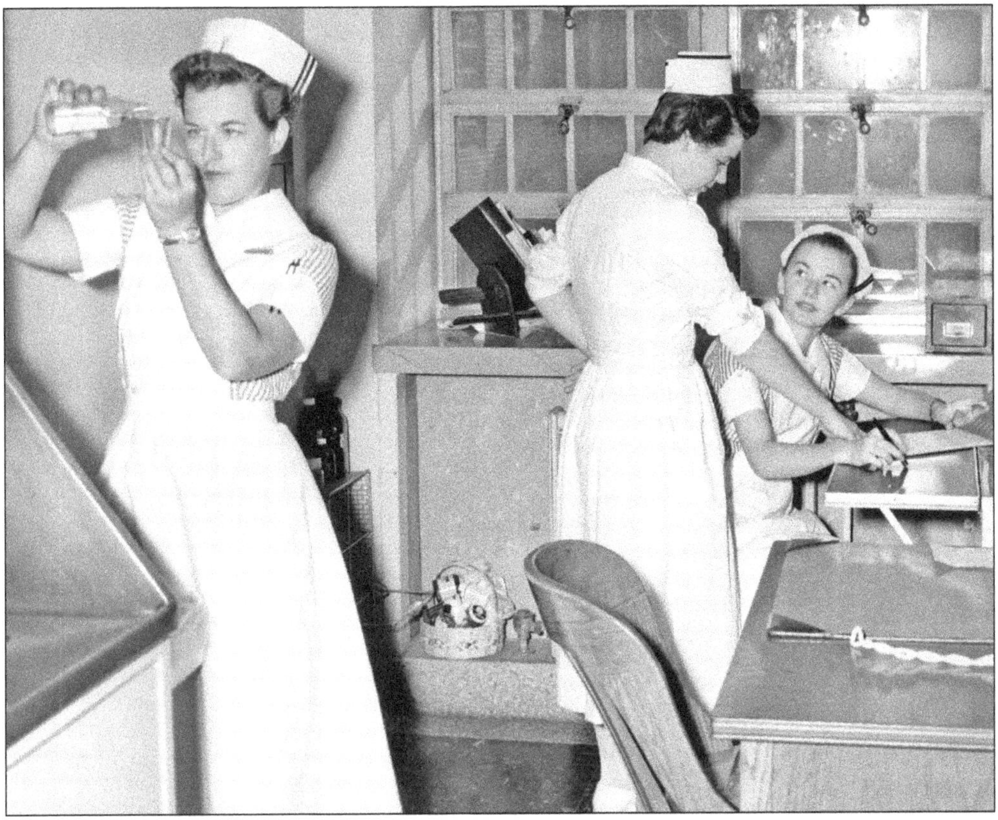

In the 1960s, compounding medication was the duty of the registered nurse under the order of the treating physician. Here, a student nurse is measuring liquid medication for a patient to ingest. A "medication cocktail" or combination of drugs would be given in liquid form, likened in jest to the cocktail one would find at a bar.

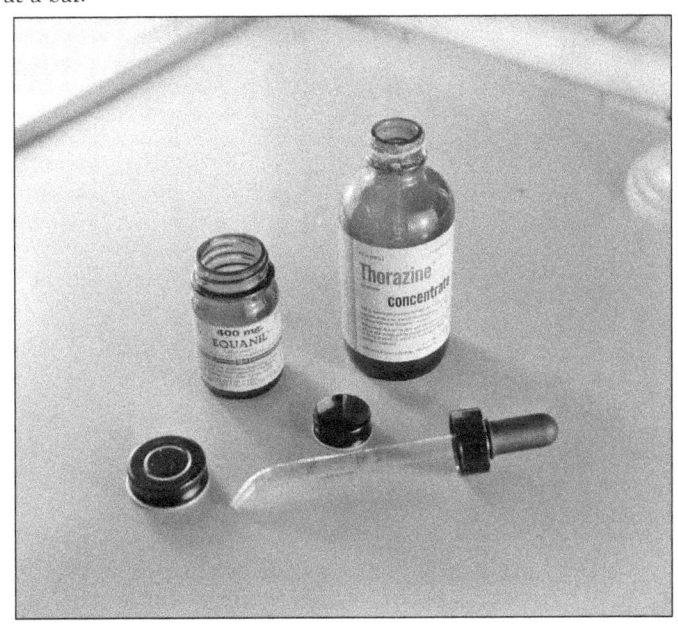

This image taken in the 1960s exhibits Thorazine, a brand name for the phenothiazine-based medication of chlorpromazine. This was the first generation of antipsychotics and the choice of the day until cloazaril was invented in the late 1980s. Discovered by accident while researchers were investigating an antihistamine medication, Thorazine was marketed to institutions as a "tranquilizing agent." In later years, the drug was given in pill form rather than liquid.

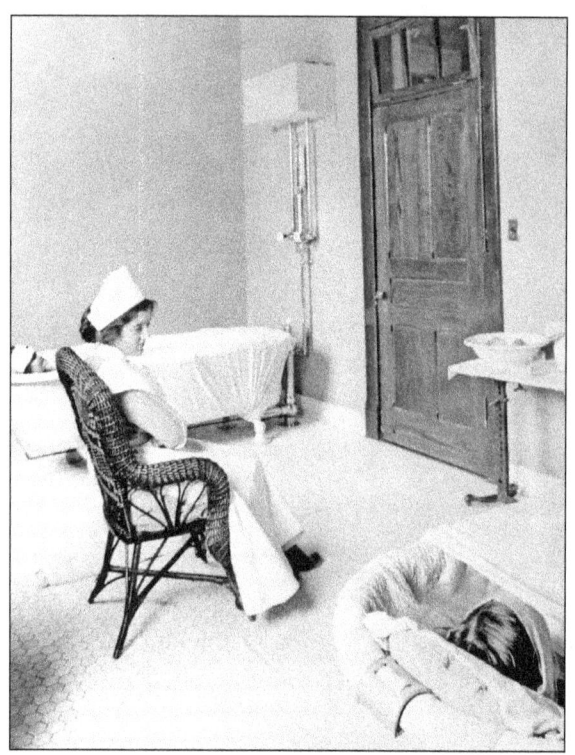

Tremendously utilized before the advent of psychotropic medication in disorders such as anxiousness, hydrotherapy was a somatic treatment. Canvas sheets were placed over the tub of warm water for privacy and to retain heat. Patients could spend hours in these tubs and were even served meals in them. Essentially, they were an early Jacuzzi, one of the only treatments with no conceivable averse side effects whatsoever.

In later years from the previous photograph, a nurse is shown here around 1950 drawing a hydrotherapy bath. Careful attention was paid to reaching a comfortable water degree for this therapy. Hydrotherapy was a responsibility the nursing staff carried out at a physician's order.

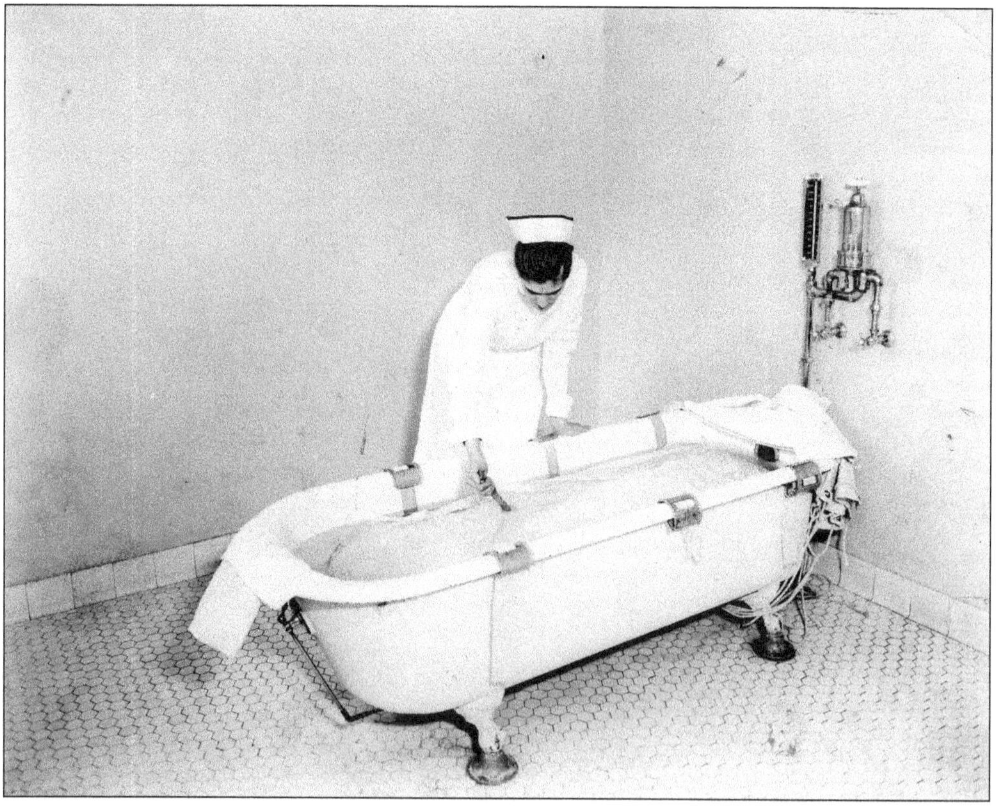

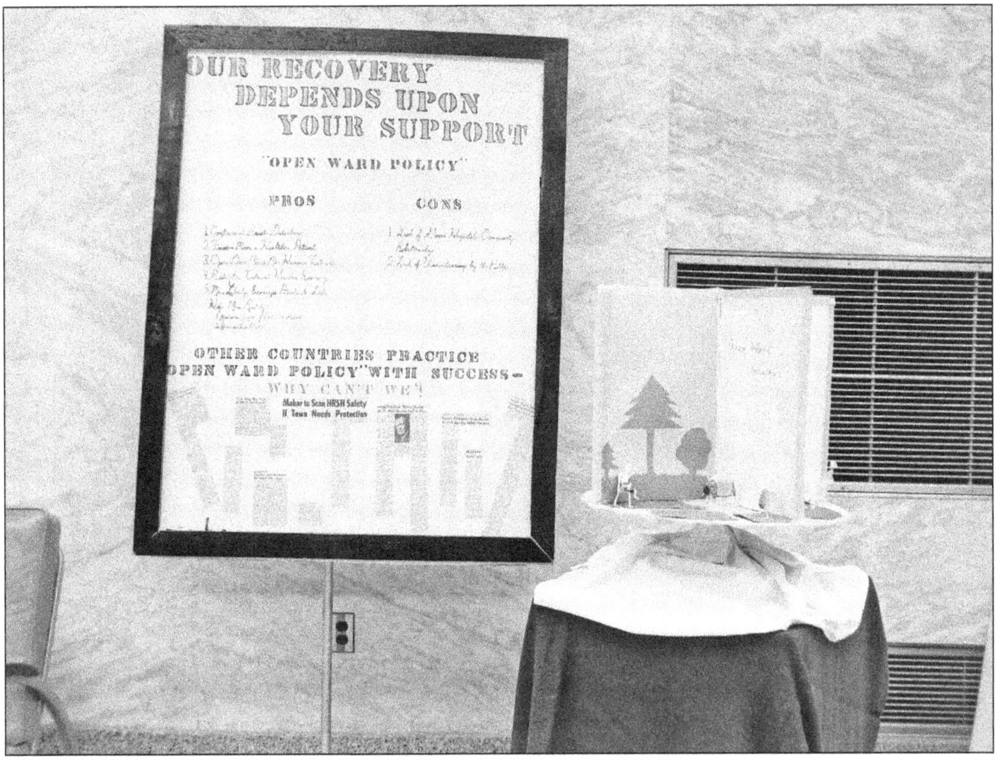

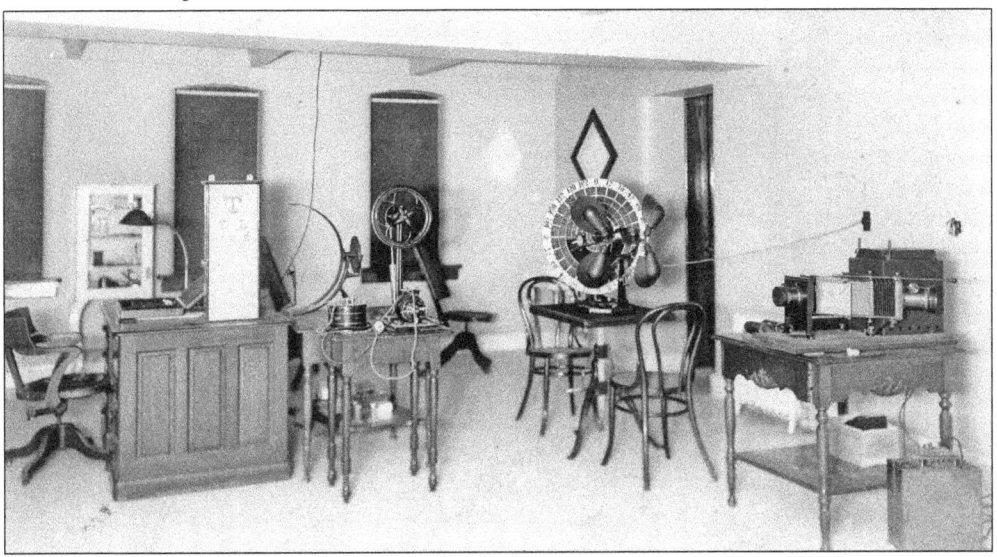

Hudson River Psychiatric Center was a leader in the 1960s under director Herman B. Snow for an "open ward policy". This referred to units being left unlocked during program hours of the day for patients to freely move through the building or grounds, depending on privilege level. In the 1960s, almost 90 percent of the wards at Hudson River were considered open wards.

During admission to the hospital, patients were examined for sight or hearing impairments. This early-1900s photograph taken in the main building shows one of the earlier examination rooms for such a purpose. As part of a yearly physical, patients were also reexamined for any new related conditions.

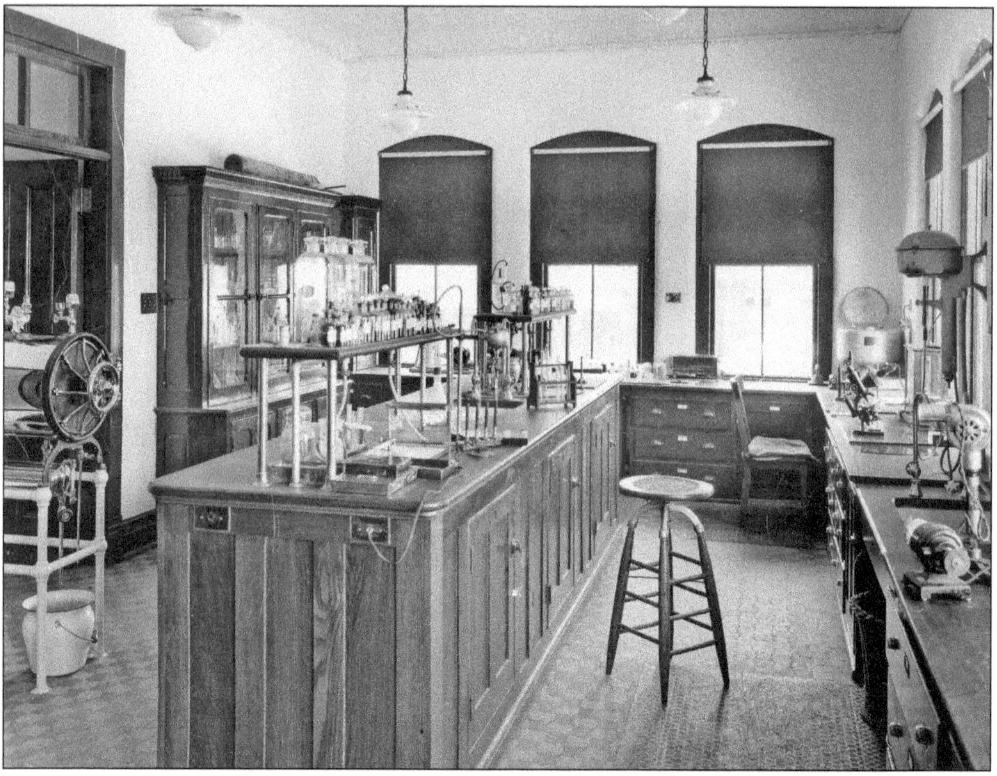

In the late 19th century, there was a new and heavy interest in the physical elements of mental disease. The pathology department at Hudson River did not only study mental disease but was also highly interested in physical illness. This state-of-the-art lab, pictured in the 1890s, did not only serve the morgue facilities in autopsy and research. Blood samples were sent here for typing and tuberculosis analysis or throat cultures for bacteriology. The lab was in the recently opened morgue and lab building behind the main building. Lab facilities for testing biological samples of the living would eventually be moved into Cheney building.

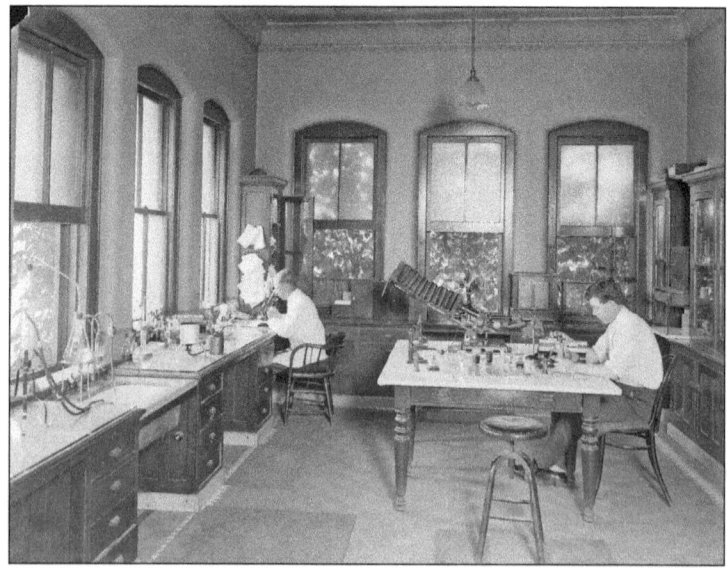

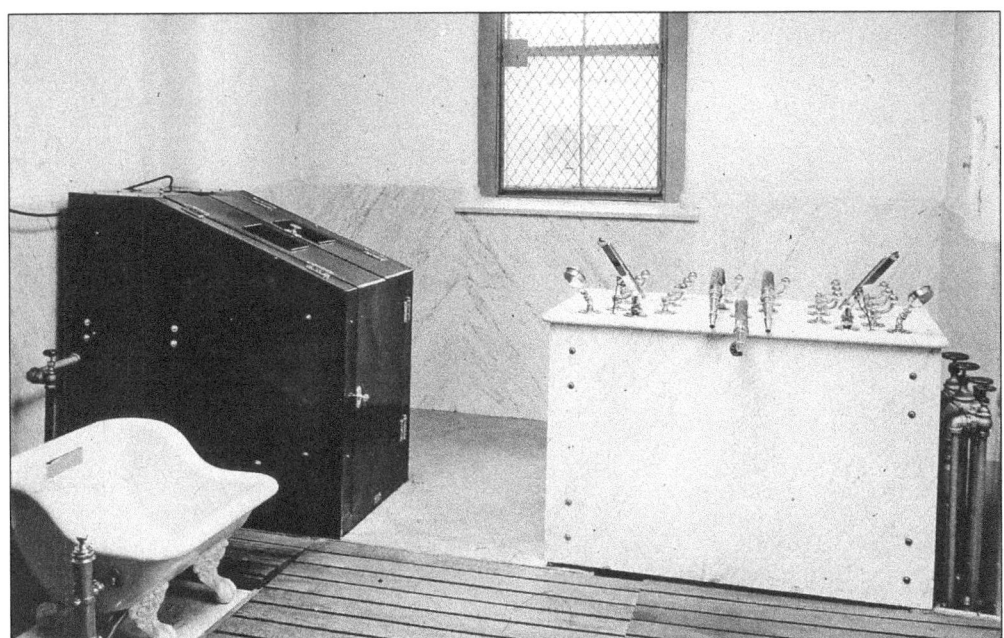

This image taken in Pilgrim Hall in the 1930s shows a large black box to the left. This was a light therapy unit. Filled with around 150 ultraviolet light bulbs, this was another somatic treatment utilized with depressed patients. Although out of use for almost 50 years, current research in depression treatment is again looking at the relation of UV light in ameliorating depression symptoms.

Delivering medical treatments as effectively and comfortably as possible to patients was of foremost importance to staff. This 1950s photograph shows an attendant modeling a simple brace device. This was used by older and feeble patients who could not hold their arm straight long enough for blood transfusions.

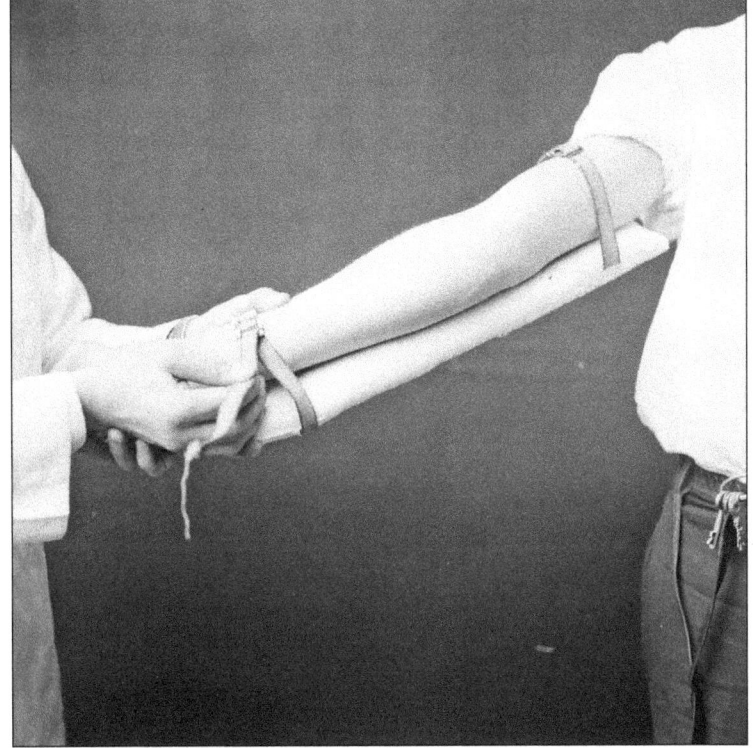

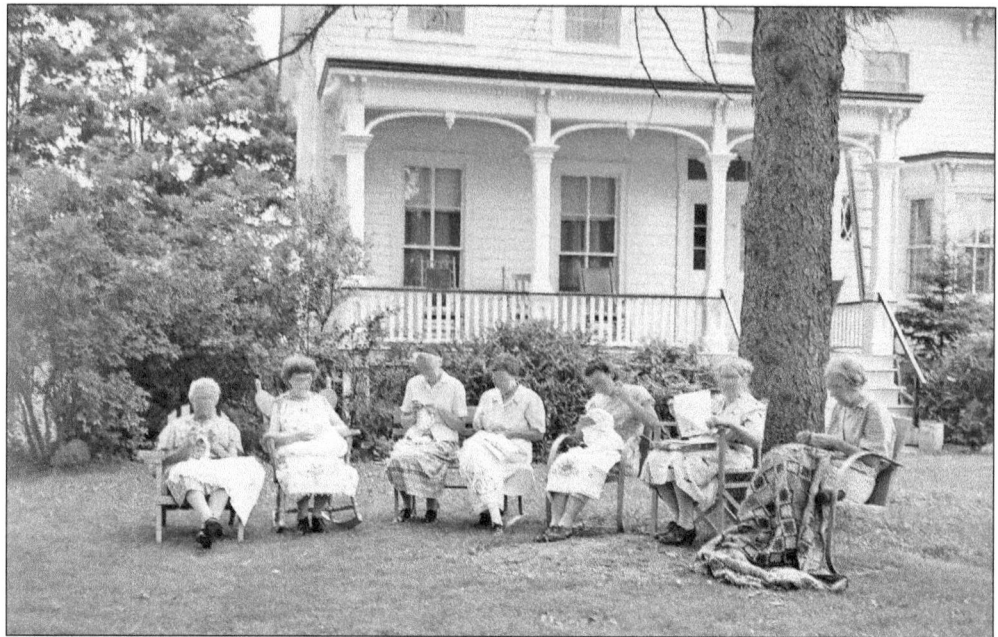

Some individuals did not require hospitalization on an inpatient unit but still needed support to move towards independent living. Skill development and training such as budgeting, self-care activities, and healthy recreational activities were taught. Small cottages that were unlocked at all times existed to house a dozen or so patients of the same sex in a transitional living setting. This cottage is one such at the hospital in the spring of 1952. Patients lived here with very few restrictions other than being inside for an established curfew and engaging in some mental health activities. Programs today run on the former Hudson River property are similar to this one, filled with individuals discharged from an inpatient facility.

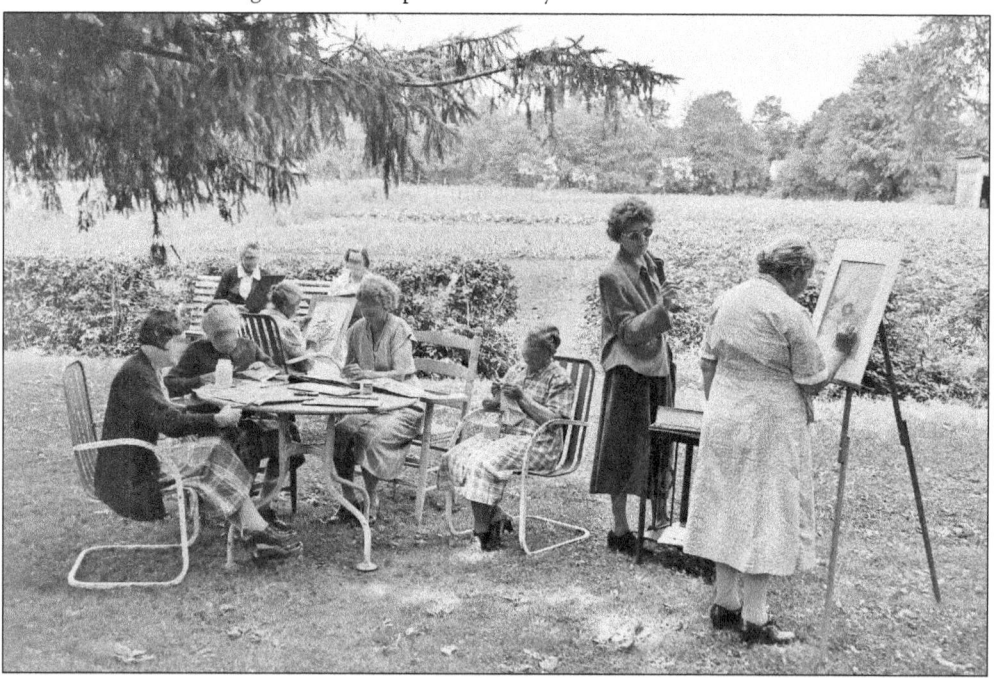

Four

FIRE AND POLICE

Fire protection has long been a concern for any facility designed for the housing and overnight lodging of any large group of individuals. Especially in the early days of the hospital before automobiles, it would be an unduly long time before aid could arrive from the Poughkeepsie Fire Department. As a result, a fire department was formed early on at Hudson River. It was not uncommon to call for mutual aid from nearby firehouses if a large-scale fire broke out. Initially, a horse-drawn pump and ladder rig was purchased. As time went on, this was replaced several times over with motorized engines. Hudson River also had its own hospital police and watchmen initially. Duties ranged from enforcing employee regulations to investigations, vehicle and traffic enforcement, and security services. Eventually, fire and police services were combined to one job function under the title of safety officer, still existent today. As active firefighting services dwindled because of modern response times from local agencies, the fire service role of the safety department vanished. In its place, a more preventative role was born in the form of officers inspecting conditions to limit risk of fire more regularly.

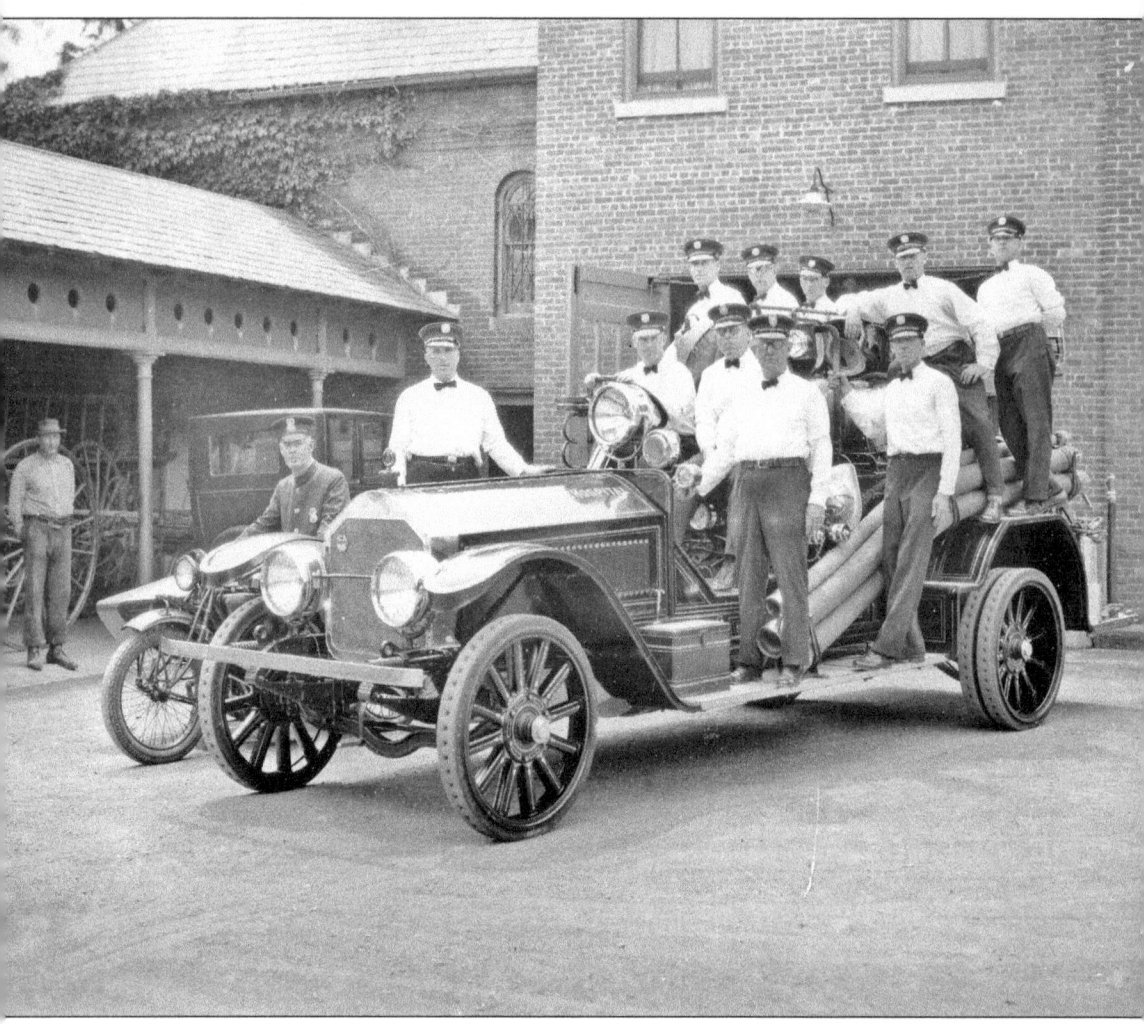

To the rear of the main building, along with trades shops, sat the fire and police building. This 1925 image shows the hospital's hook and ladder truck along with the men of the fire department. On board were hand-operated ladders, pike poles (used to pull down plaster ceilings during a fire), axes, and the other necessary tools of the trade to fight a fire. The truck also had buckets that could be filled with water and brought to a fire, a variety of hose lengths, and a water can extinguisher. As technology advanced, engines would be capable of carrying hundreds of gallons of onboard water, unlike this truck, which carried none. To the left, a hospital policeman sits on his patrol motorcycle. Under the awning sit the ladders used by the firemen for rescue and firefighting.

Although the hospital was not what most people would consider a high-traffic area, it was not without automobile accidents. This image taken behind the main building, near the storehouse, shows a car that collided with the railroad signal. Accident investigations such as this were dealt with by the hospital police in the safety department.

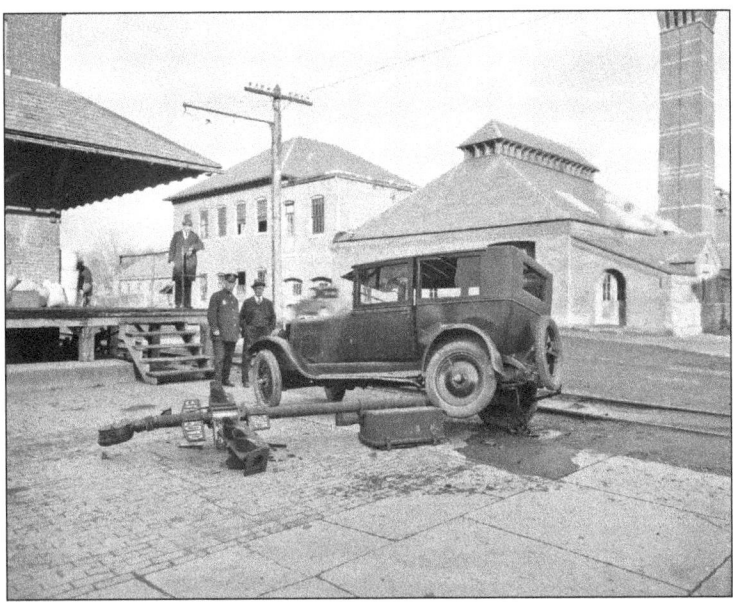

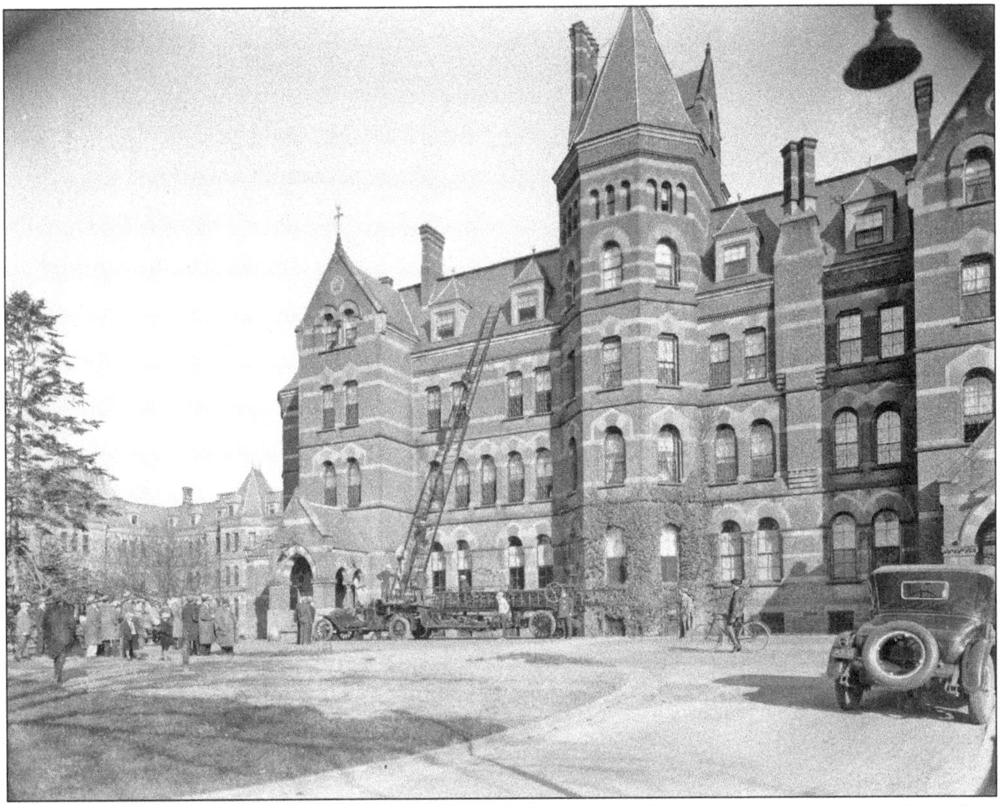

Being prepared for any arising fire-related emergency was the duty of the men in the safety department. Rigorous training on all the hospital buildings was a regular occurrence to keep fire fighters well trained and ready to respond. This 1950s image shows the hospital firemen and Poughkeepsie Fire Department preforming a drill together on a ladder truck. Spectators watch the men climb the ladder up the face of the building.

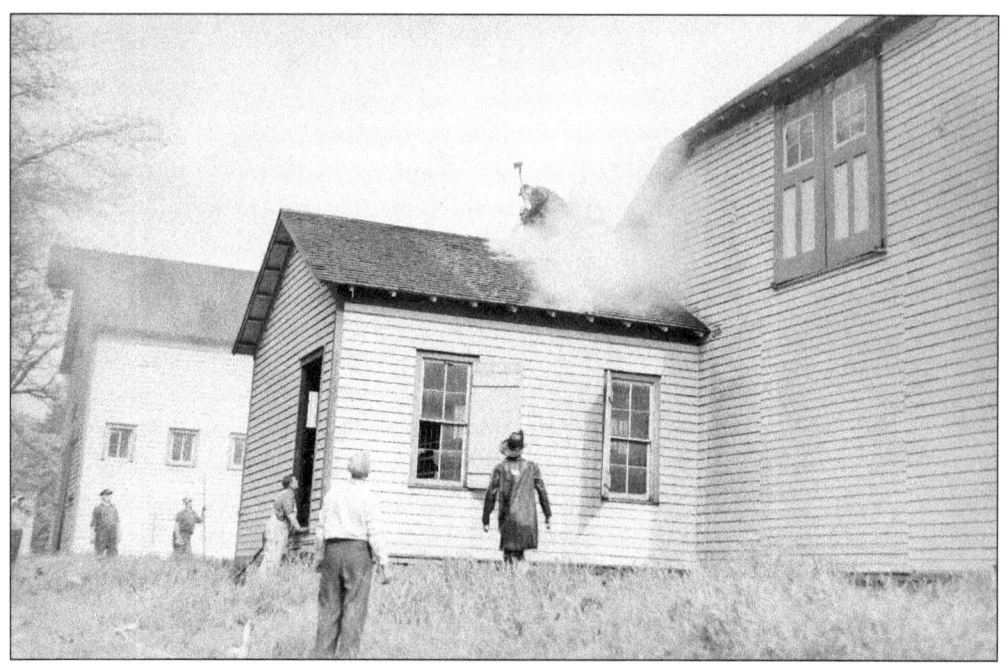

As time went on, buildings' purposes changed, including this barn. Originally part of the hospital farm, this later became used for housing transportation vehicles. This photograph, taken in May 1955, shows a fire at the barn. On the roof, a fireman can be seen axing a vent into the roof to release smoke from the interior.

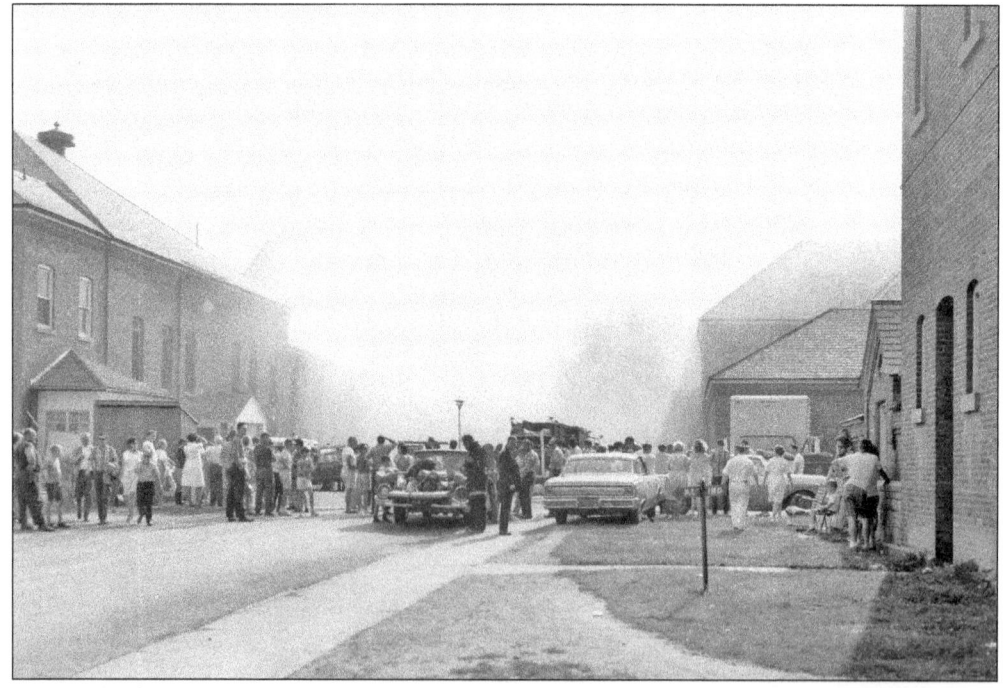

Smoke fills the background of this 1971 photograph taken behind the main building. A fire broke out towards the rear of the patient wards, close to the shops. In the center, a hospital fireman can be seen suited up with an air pack.

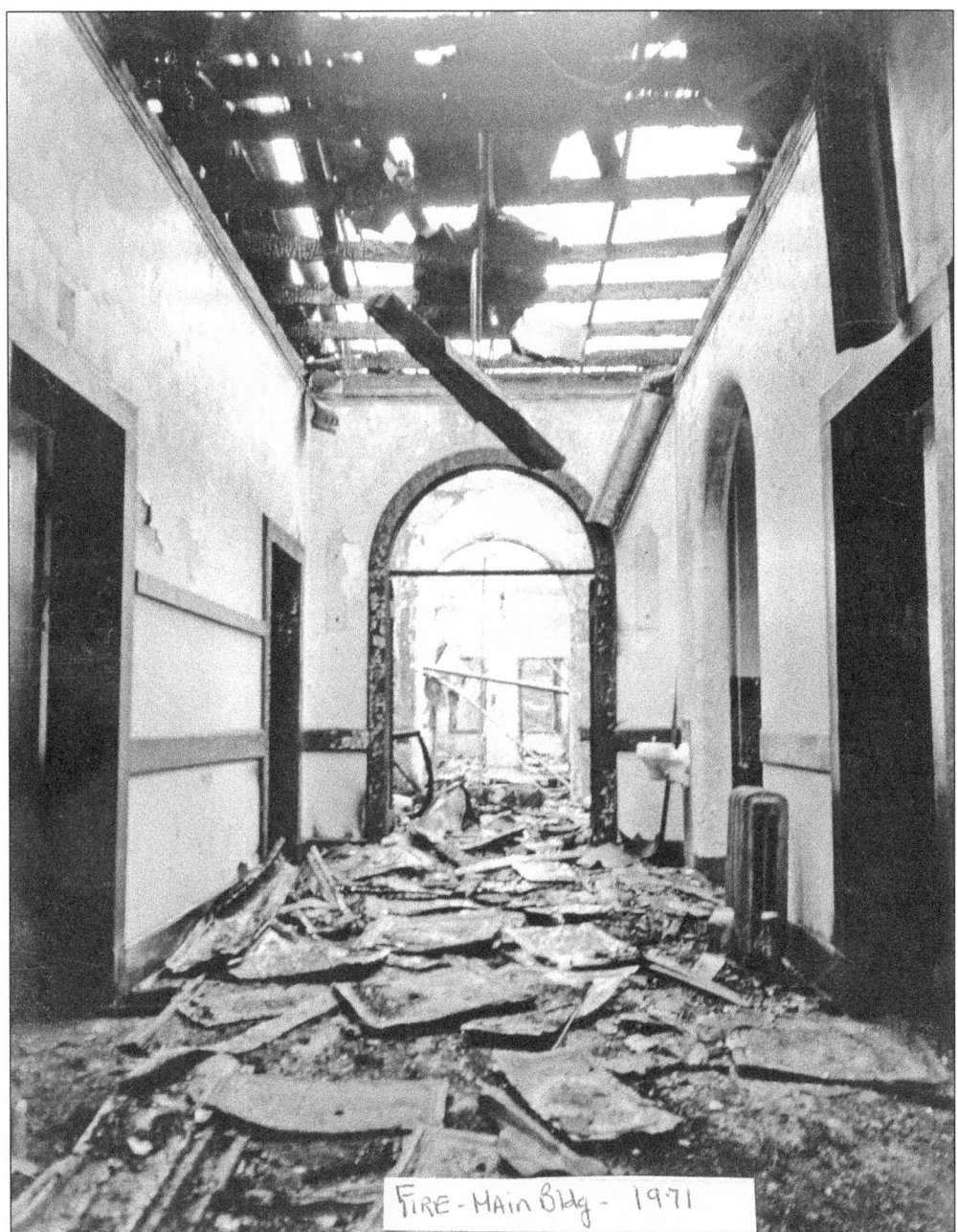

Shown here is the interior damage to the second floor in the south wing of the main building following a fire in 1971. Charred door frames and hanging electrical fixtures can be seen. Much of the ceiling remains on the floor as part of the effort to ensure the fire was extinguished fully. Although the building had a stone and brick facade, the floors and roof were entirely of wood. Fire prevention at the facility was always of extreme importance. Every staff member in the hospital, regardless of position, carried two keys in addition to all others. One key rang the fire alarm, and one key permitted exit from all buildings interiors, regardless of location. This was to prevent entrapment during a fire. This fire occurred in the daytime on a ward of the building designed for patient living; no one was injured.

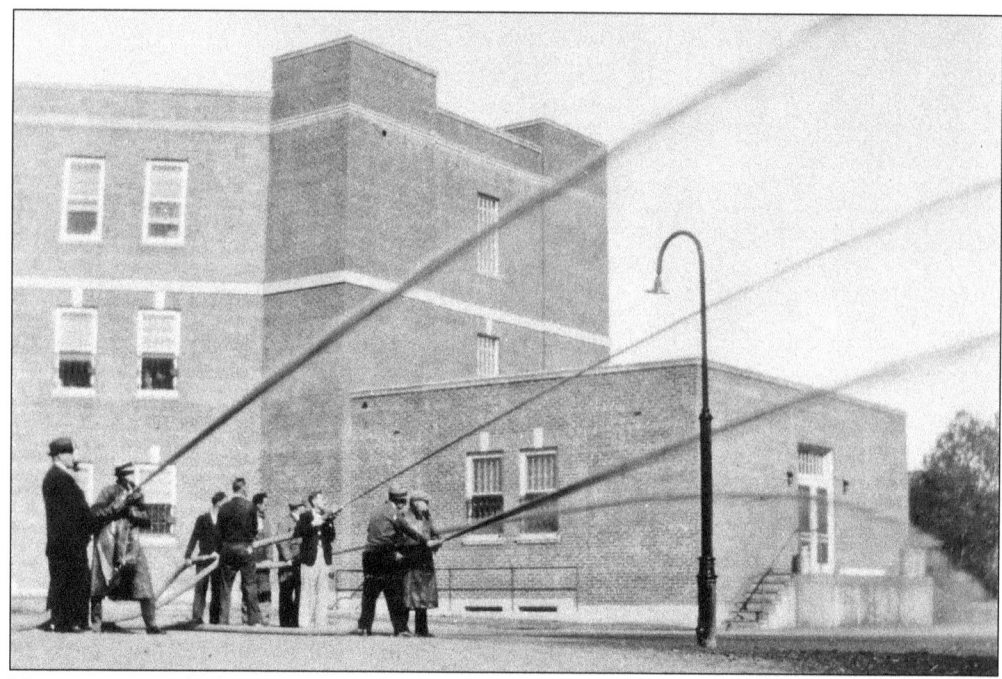

Hose operation drills were routine practice for the hospital fire department. This was to test equipment as well as to ensure familiar and fast operating of hose apparatus. This 1950s photograph was taken in the rear of Ryon Hall in the spring. From the windows, spectators watch on.

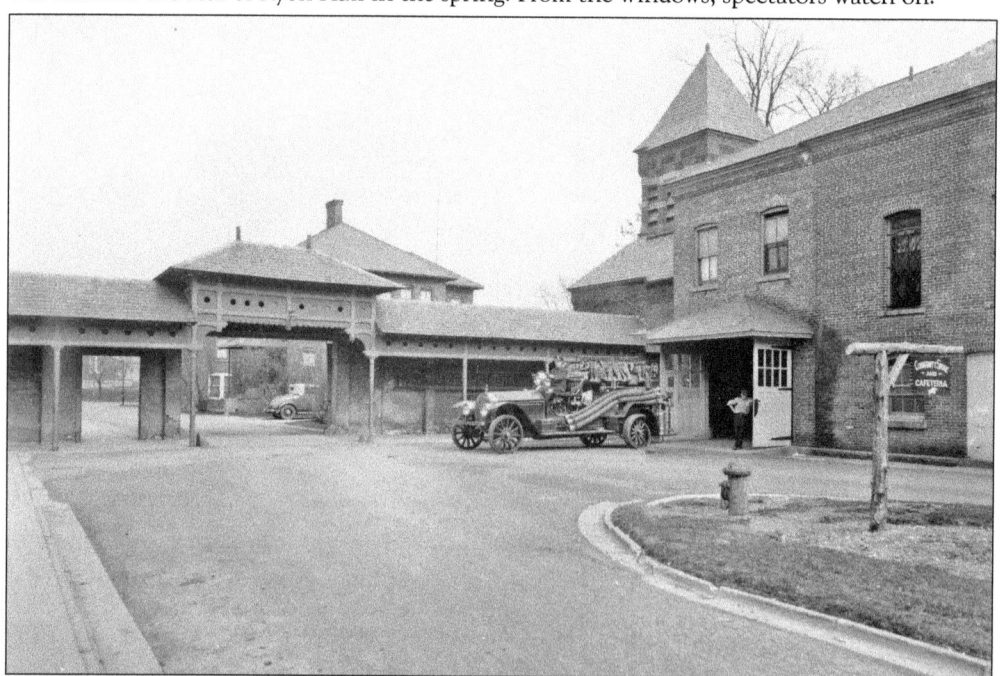

Taken with a larger angle of view, this 1920s image shows the fire truck for the hospital with its chauffeur. On board, the firemen's boots and equipment can be seen. The opening in the wall had a gate that could be closed. This formed a secure courtyard area that inpatients from the main building could use.

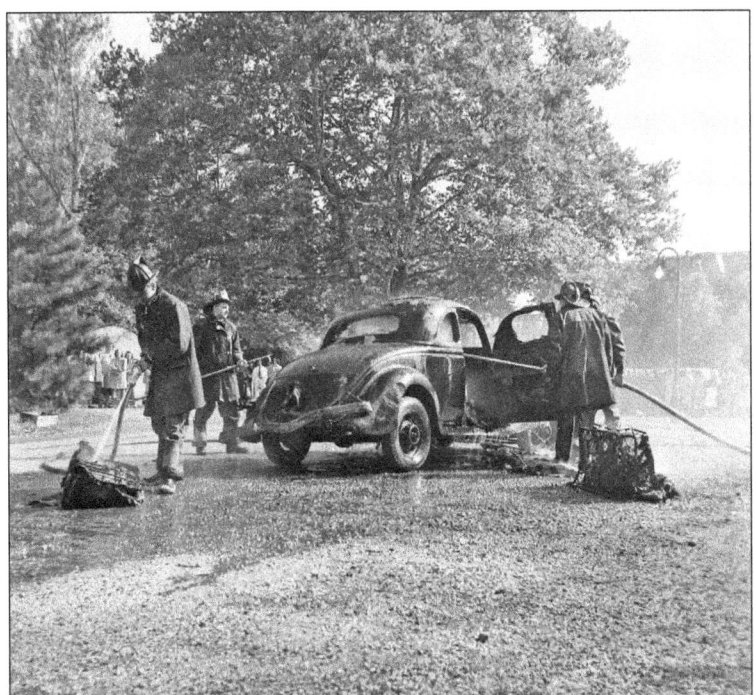

Demonstrations for staff by the hospital fire department were not an overly regular sight. Here a live burn demonstration at Hudson River takes place outside the main building in October 1952. In the background, dozens of individuals are shown huddled about watching the firefighting. In a large lodging facility, it was critical to stress fire safety practice to all staff and patients.

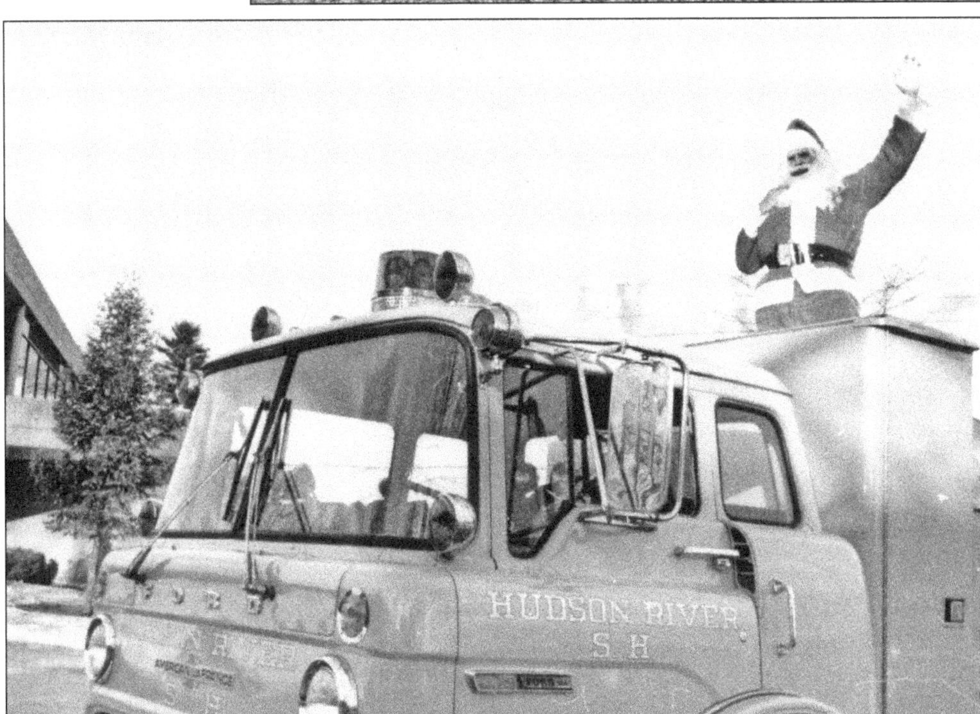

Outside of being first responders, fire trucks were a familiar sight at the hospital during Christmas. In this 1970s photograph, Santa can be seen outside Snow Rehab building riding along in the truck. Securing a cheerful environment for the patients at the hospital, especially on the holidays, was taken seriously by all staff.

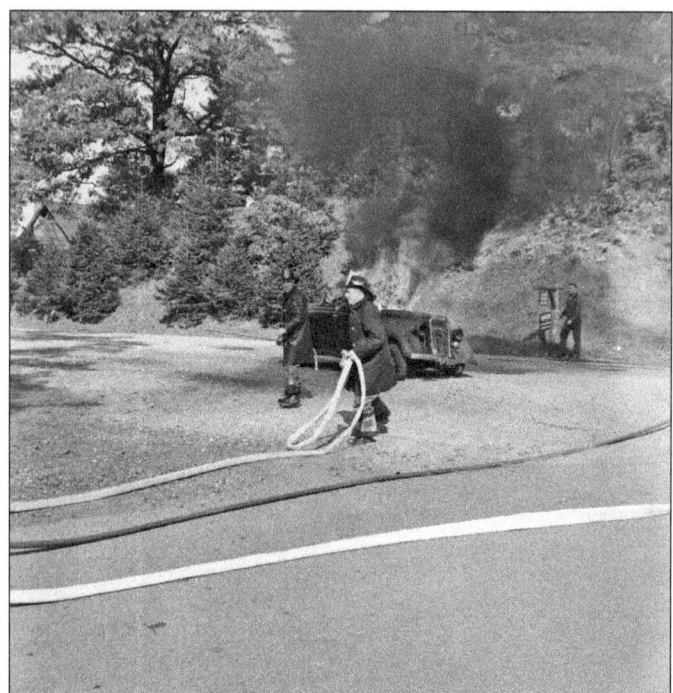

Practice drills with various fire materials and scenarios were part of an ongoing training program. In order to be prepared for the many circumstances that could be encountered in a fire incident at the hospital, keeping firefighting skills sharp was imperative. In these images, Hudson River's fire department is seen practicing extinguishing simulated live burn fires.

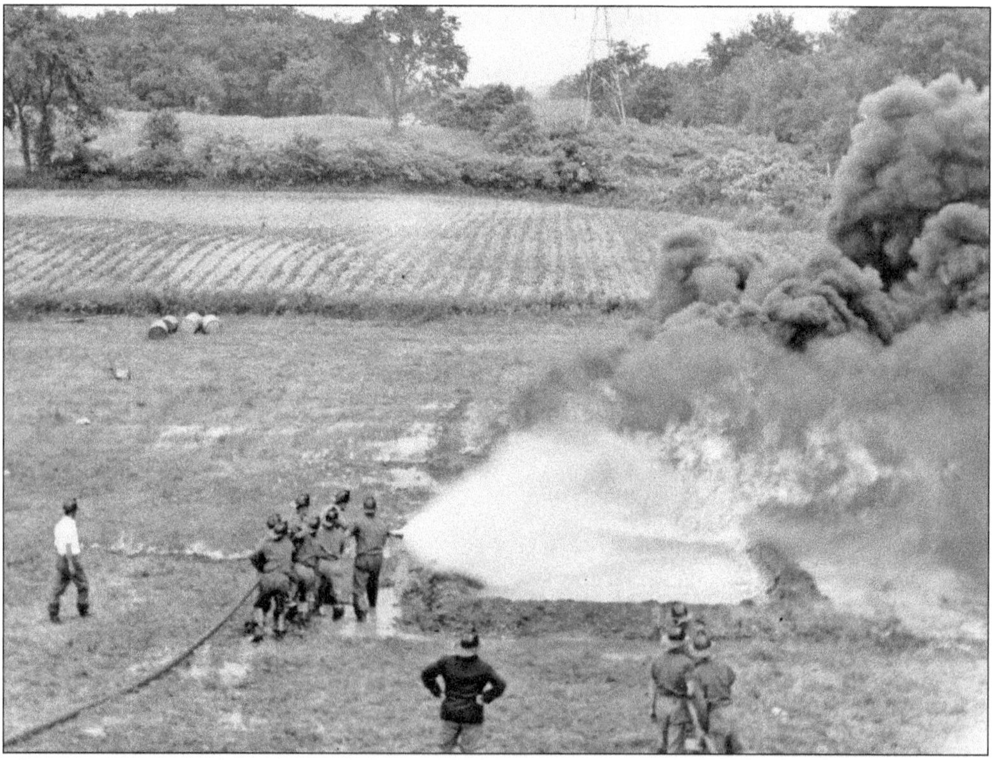

The image taken in the field is a drill with the local Fairview Fire Department. The car fire drill (pictured) was conducted on the grounds of the hospital near the main building. In more serious building fires, aid from all surrounding fire service agencies was called in for additional recourses.

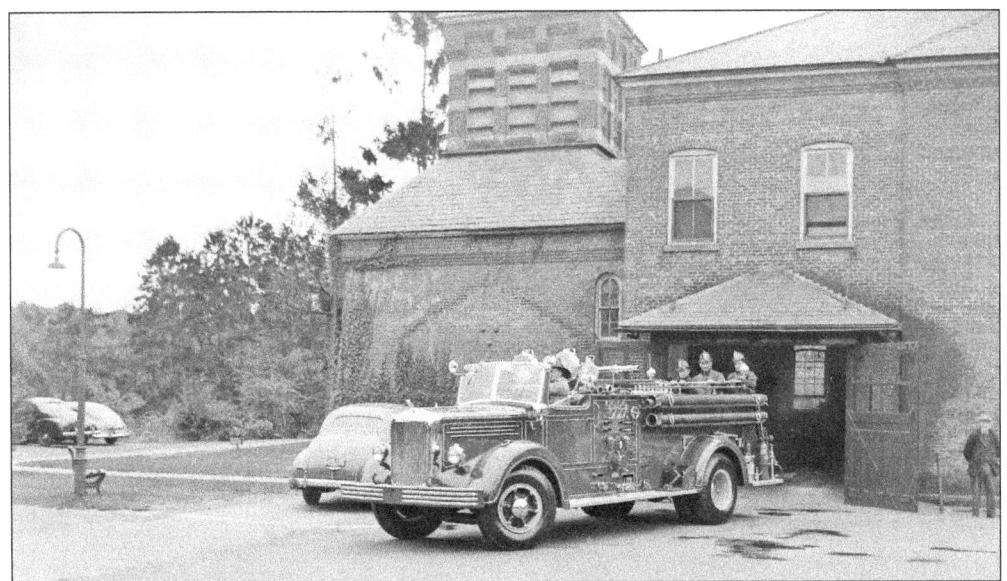

Above, in 1951 the hospital's engine is seen leaving the garage. Unlike earlier trucks at Hudson River, this rig was equipped with onboard water in order to extinguish a fire without immediate hydrant access. Because of the many wooden structures on the grounds at the time, a fast response was critical in the event of a structure fire at the hospital. The men in the photograph are traveling to a fire drill on the grounds. Below, the same truck can be seen in use during a drill with several of the hospital firemen.

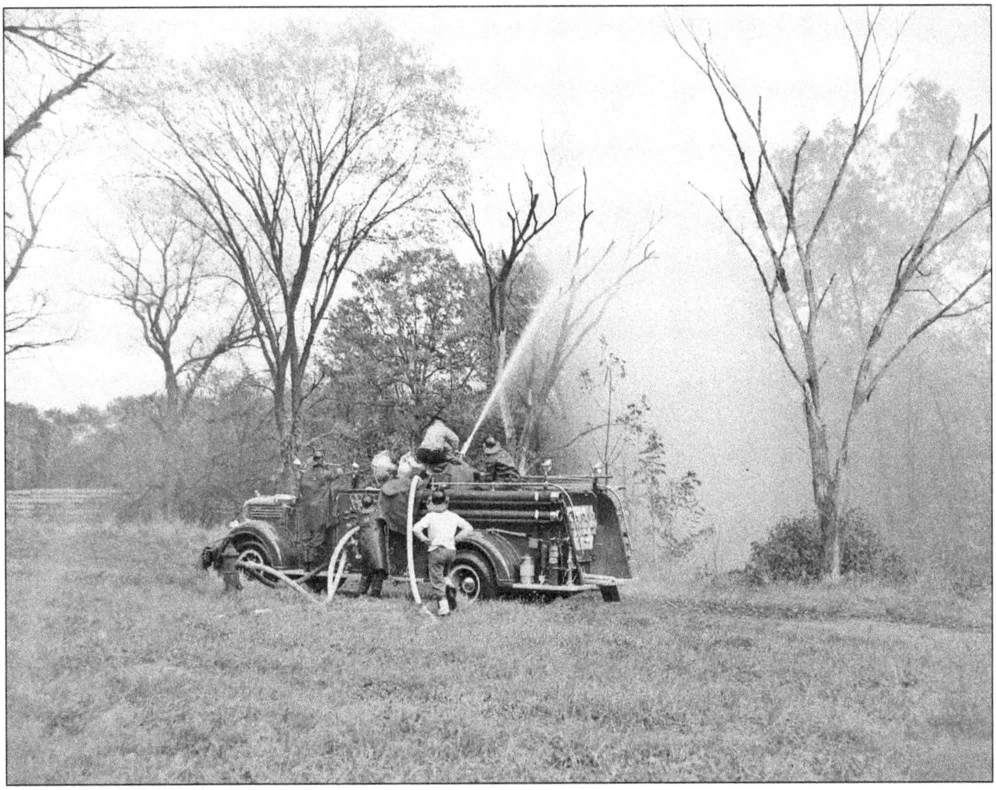

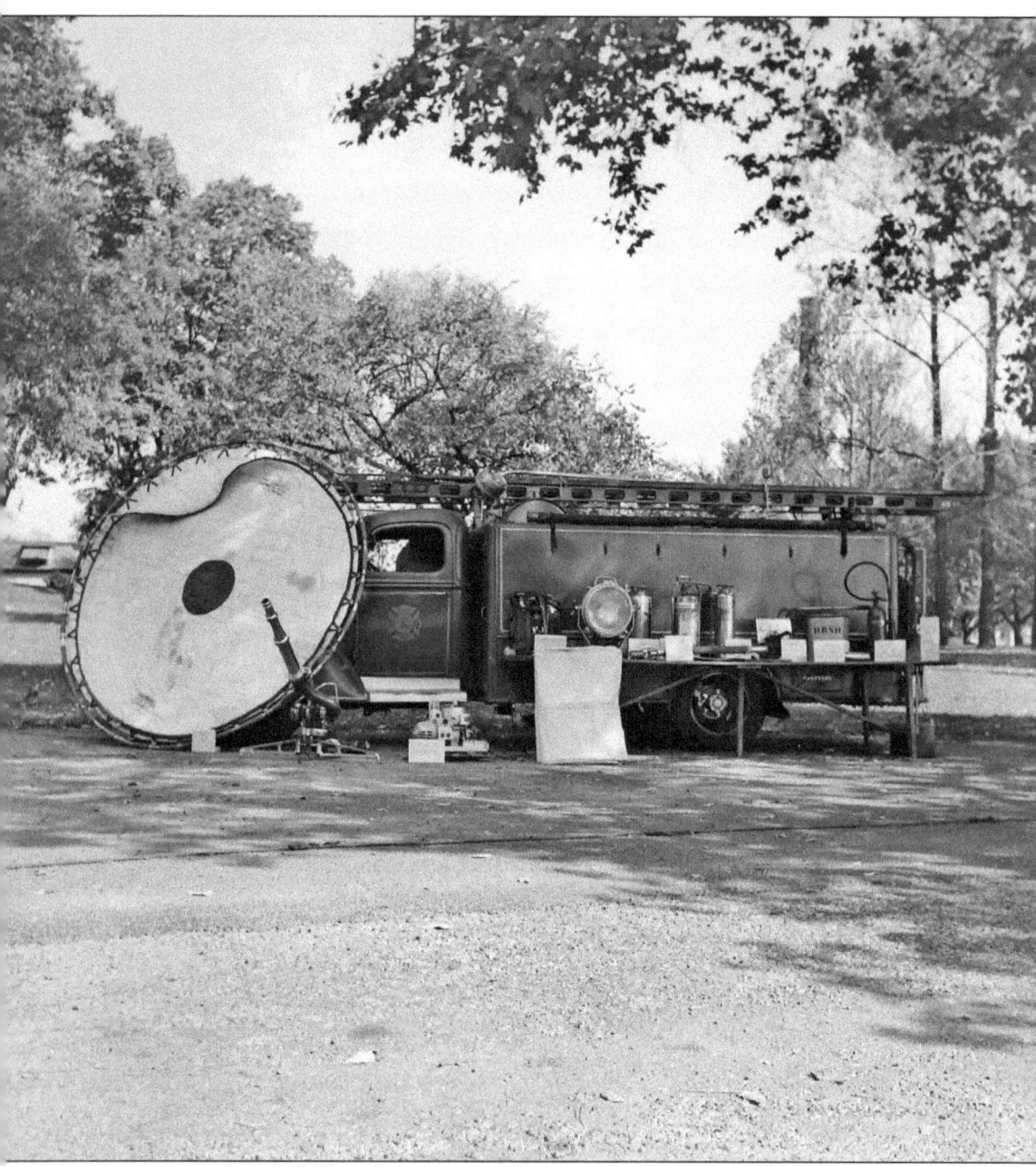

This 1952 photograph shows the hospital fire truck and some of the common tools of the trade at the time. To the left stands a large cloth circle with a bull's-eye. This was used to catch individuals who need to jump out a window or off a roof in a fire emergency. This was an especially useful technique in the event of a blaze on a ward with many occupants. This allowed evacuation to happen quicker than dozens of people climbing down a ladder. In the days before Cheney Memorial, there were no structures higher than four stories, and this could be used at all of the buildings. To promote fire awareness and safety, exhibits were displayed for the staff by the safety department. This photograph was taken on the grounds during one such exhibit.

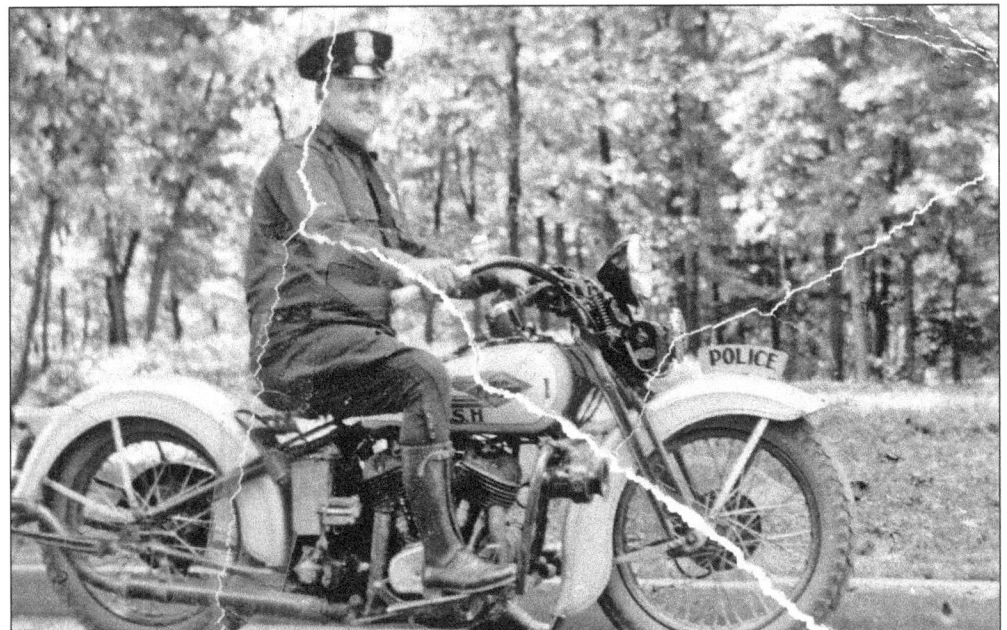

Although a bit tattered, this 1920s photograph features a hospital policeman. If one looks closely at his leg, the "S.H" in "H.R.S.H" can be made out. Above the front tire would have sat a red light for use in his duties as a police officer. A small siren can be spotted to the rear of the front fender as well.

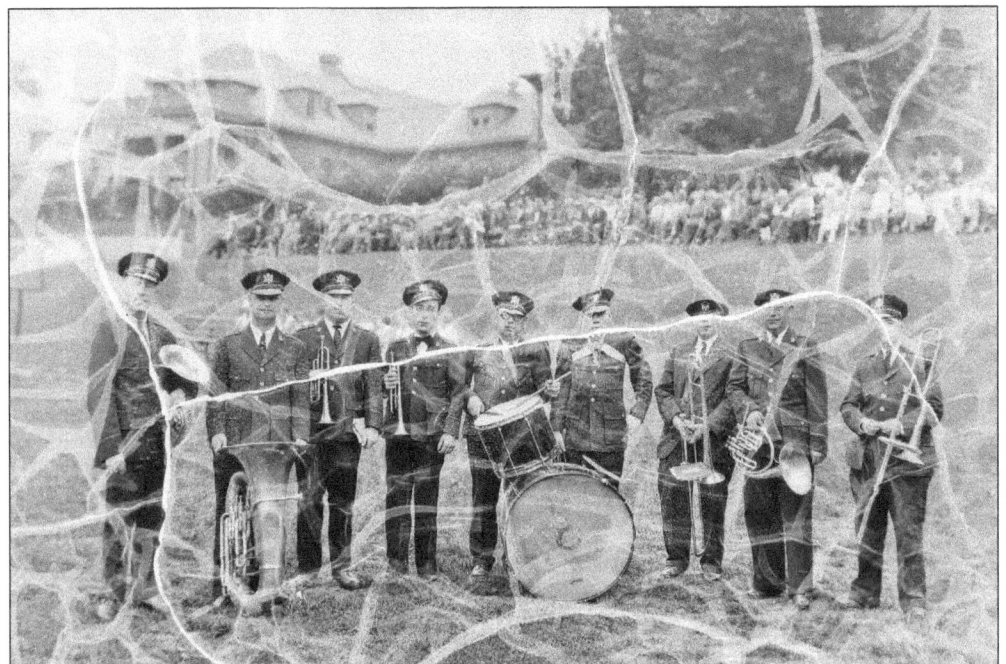

Outside of fire and police services, this 1950s image shows another faculty of the safety department. Here at a field day celebration, the fire- and policemen play a tune for the staff and patients of the hospital. The class A dress uniform worn here was far more formal than the everyday uniform these men would wear.

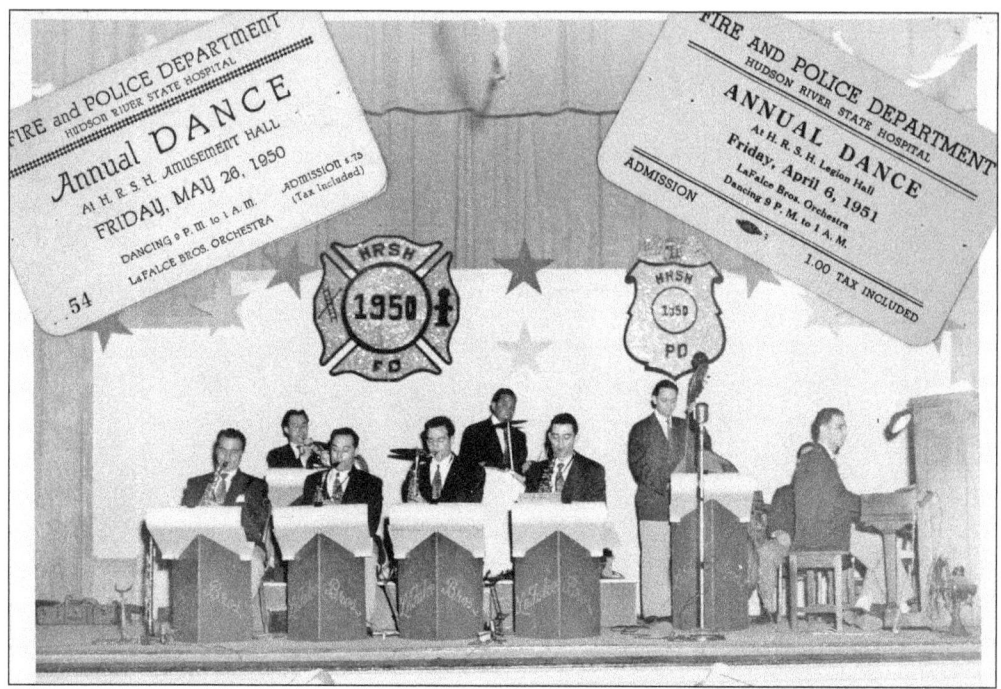

Aside from working closely together in the same department, the men and women of the safety department shared many social functions. This police and fire dance in 1950 is an example of such a social gathering. Family members, friends, and spouses were welcome to join these gatherings. Above is a 75¢ admission ticket to the dance.

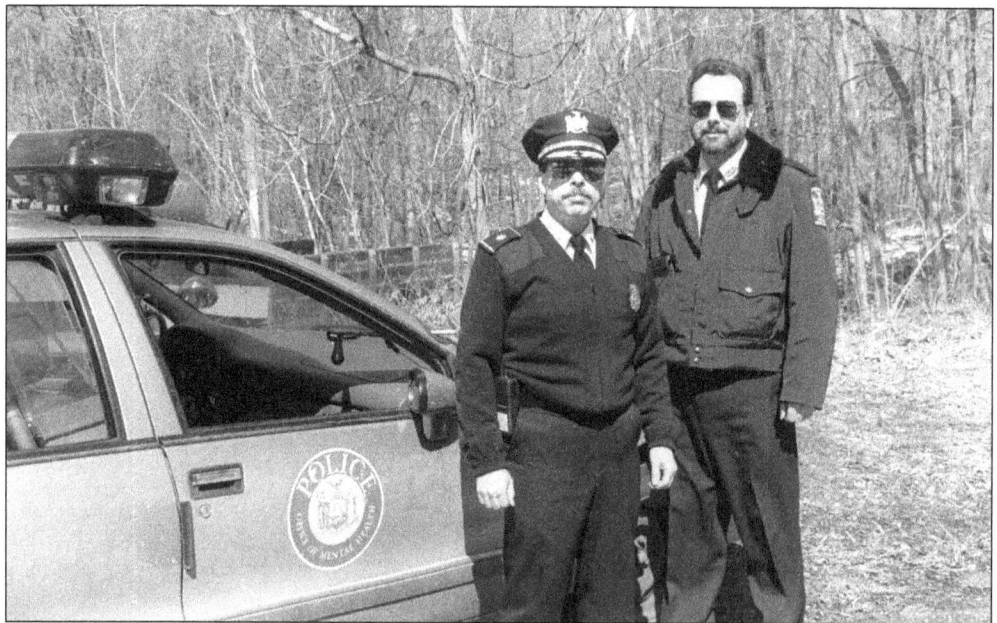

This 1990s photograph shows one of the last chiefs of the safety department at Hudson River and one of his officers. Chief Nick Cuomo (left) and an Officer Peotoss are pictured outside their patrol vehicle on the grounds of the lower campus near Paint Shop Road. By the lack of leaves and their clothing, they appear to be performing their duties in early winter.

Five

THE FARMS

The farms at Hudson River played a substantial role in the autonomy, finance, and treatment at the facility. Patient labor aided work with grain, livery, and produce. As much as two thirds of the food consumed on the grounds was grown at the hospital from the 19th century through the just past the mid-20th century. Patients worked in every aspect of farming. Part of the plan for the construction of the Central Group complex was individual hamlets with farmland for each building of patients to grow food. Duties were not limed to warm weather; in winter, farmers had several charges related to ice and snow. At the hospital's peak, farm operations were certainly a foundational feature critical to its autonomous operations. Excess produce was sold in New York City markets, bringing funds to the hospital. A line of credit was established with other state hospitals, jails, and state schools for the mentally handicapped for trading grain, produce, and livery products. This credit system kept operating costs throughout the state low and ensured nothing was wasted.

In the 1960s, being federally required to pay a salary to patient workers made staffing the farms fiscally impossible. Therefore, the farms were decommissioned as a source of produce for suppling the state hospitals. In a conversation this author had with the 1960s commissioner of the Department of Mental Hygiene for New York State, Dr. Allen Miller recalled that patients from the Letchworth Village facility, a state school for the mentally handicapped in Rockland County, took buses all the way to the capital in Albany to protest the decision. Farming was much more than a source of income for patients, it was a vocation that gave them pride. Sadly, the state officials had little choice in the matter, as federal labor regulations sublated the treatment and dignity of thousands of patients in institutions around the country.

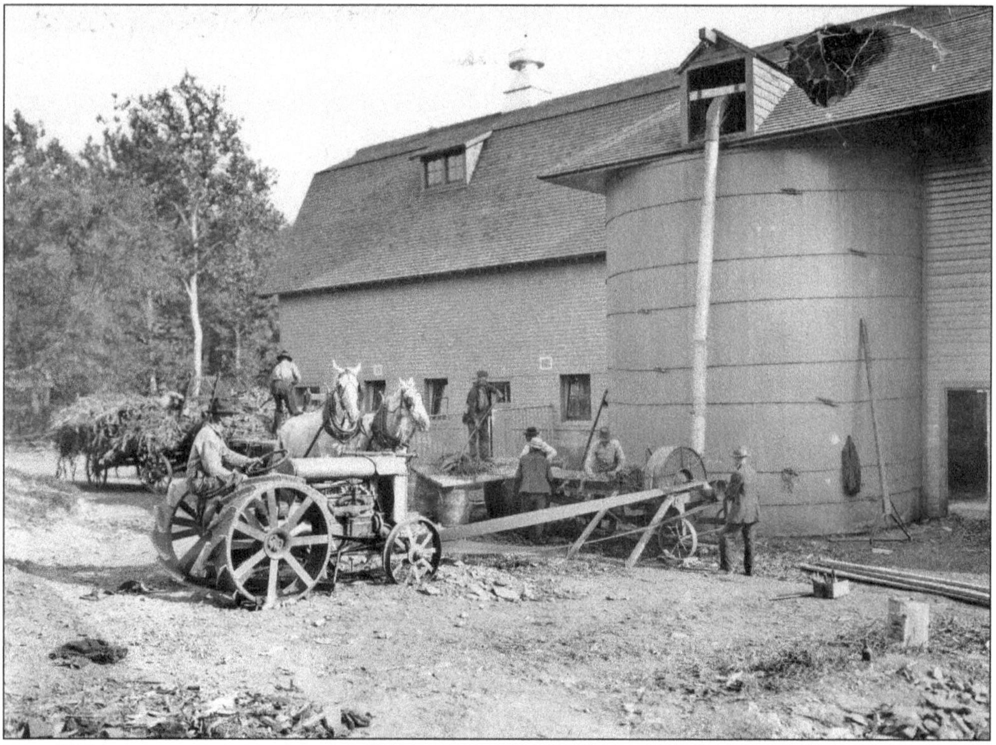

This 1920s image shows a tractor-powered hopper system for moving feed corn into storage. To the left, a horse-drawn cart of cornstalks awaits processing. A work station made of barrels and boards serves as the assembly line to transform the raw crop into usable feed for the animals at the facility.

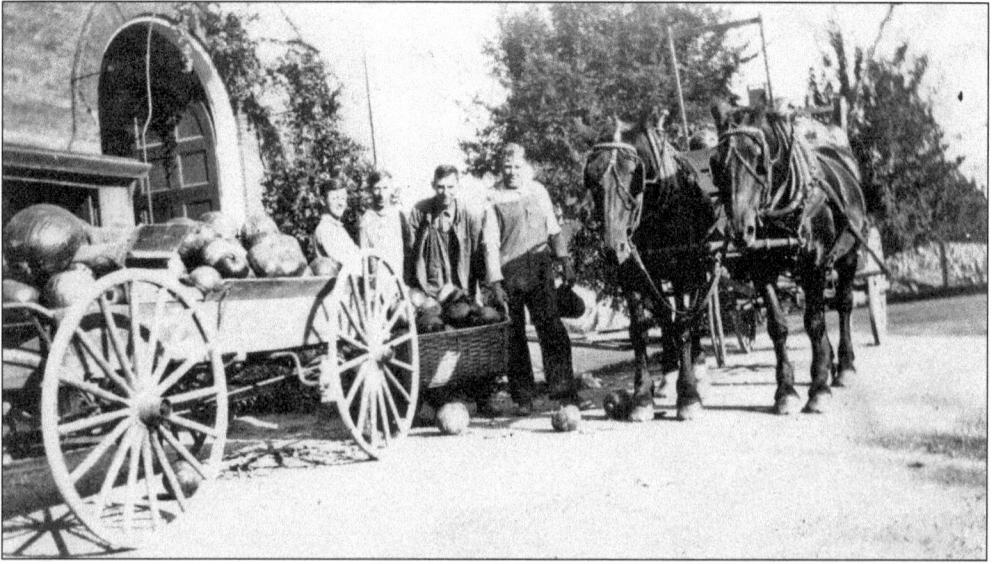

Fall harvest gave way to a number of ornamental and kitchen yields. In this image taken at the Central Group, horse-drawn flats with pumpkins can be seen. Aside from making delicious pies, the pumpkins provided decorations for the fall holidays at the hospital in full harvest spirit. Pumpkin carving could be done on the wards by the occupational therapy department at this time.

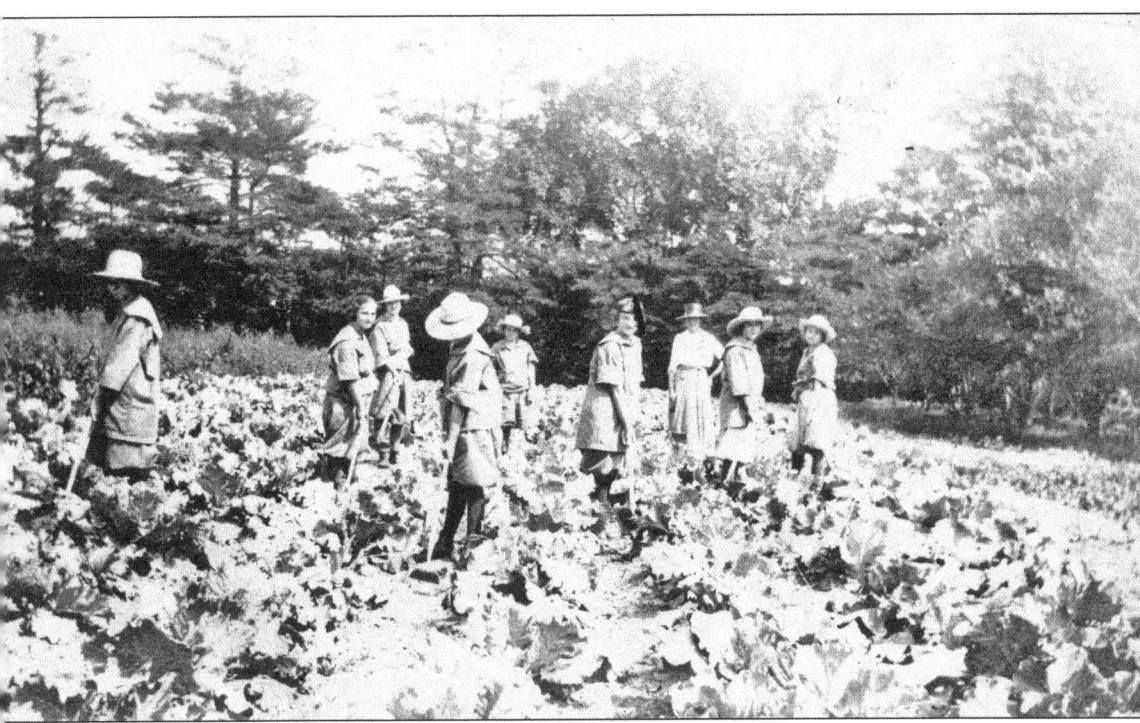

In the farm operation, men and women did not intermingle during the workday. Here, across the campus at a different farm site, women can be seen weeding a field of collard greens. It is important to note that it is hard to make the connection that some individuals are indeed patients living in a psychiatric hospital. This would be a sight no different than any other small rural farm of the day.

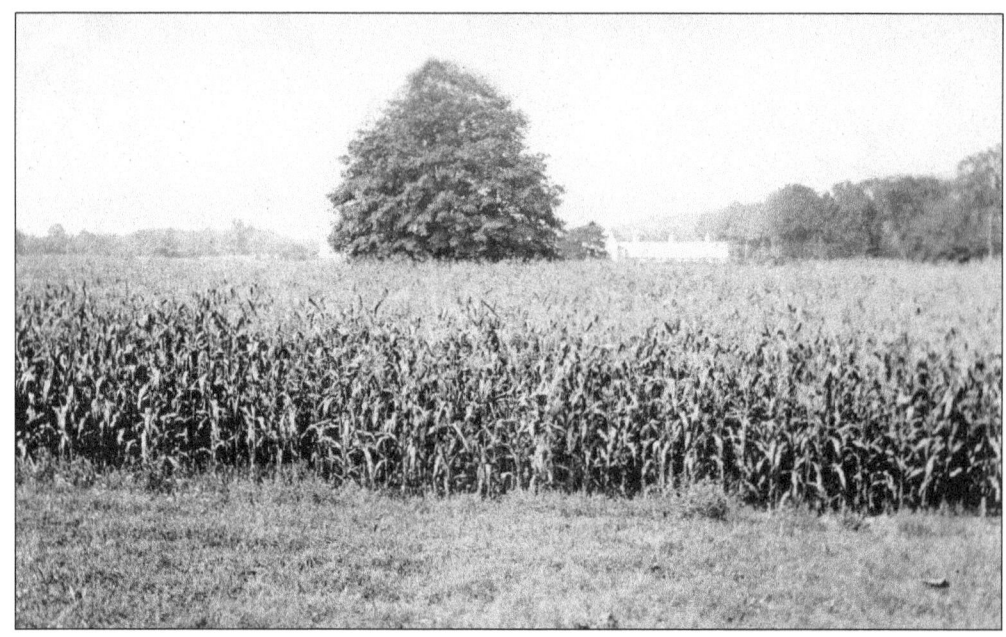

Corn dominated the farm landscape at Hudson River for many decades. Two varieties of corn were grown on grounds, feed corn for livestock and sweet corn for human consumption. With early and late summer harvests as well as a fall harvest, the yield in pounds of corn was tremendous. Above, the large cornfield to the west of the main building can be seen with the conservatory in the background at right. Below, a farmer inspects the fields on his horse and buggy. The farms shuttered in the later 1960s. For the great majority of time the farms ran at Hudson River, the farmers relied on horses for plowing, pulling material, and transportation.

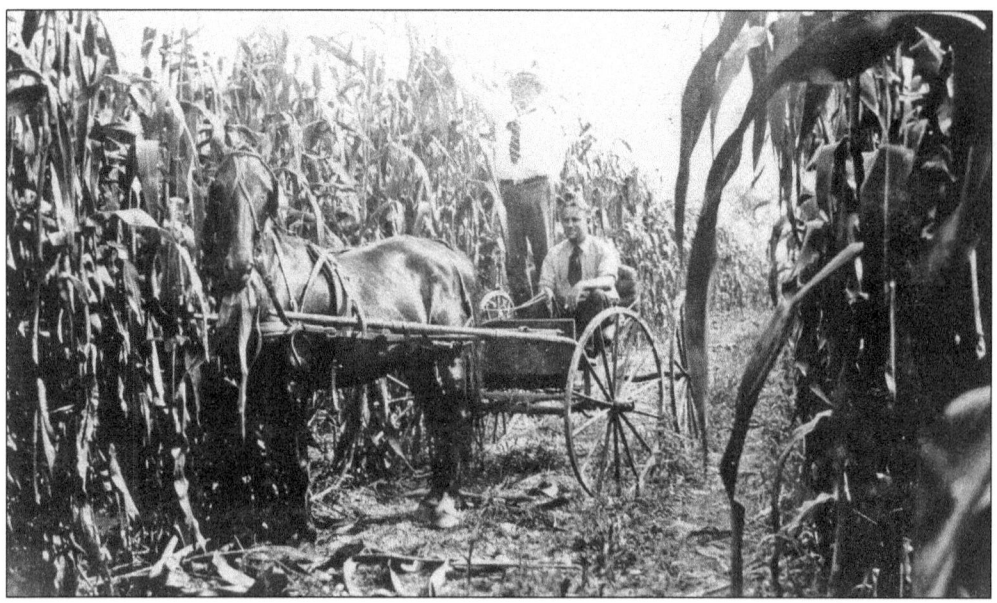

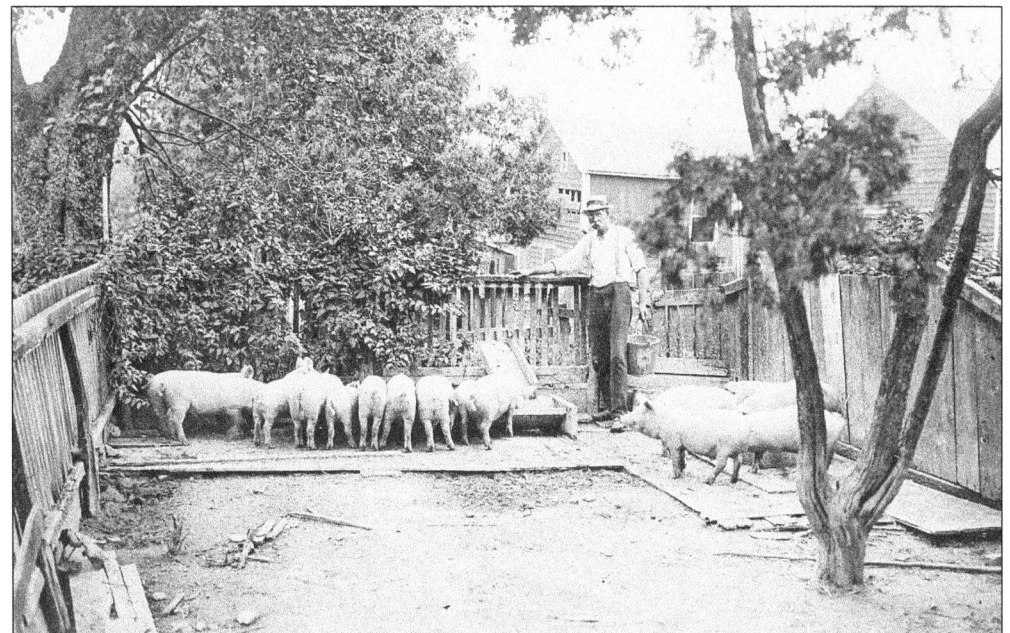

The hospital was equipped with a piggery, which raised large numbers of pigs for slaughter. Pigs were economic to raise, as they were often fed leftover meals that would have gone to waste otherwise. In this image, men working at the piggery proudly display some of their prize hogs for the year.

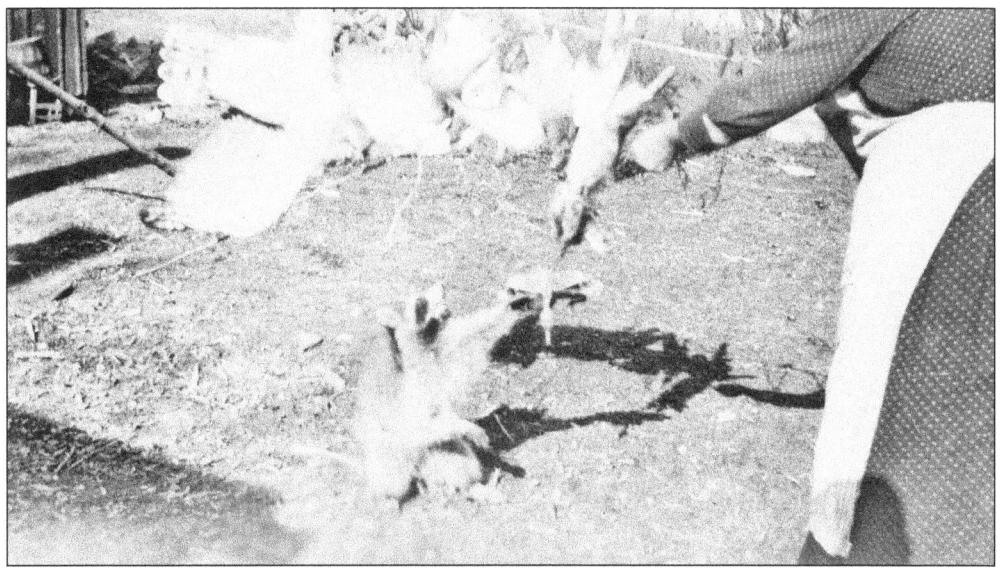

Foul was raised on the farm as well in its heyday. Chickens are shown being prepared to be defeathered. In addition to birds to be used in the kitchen, a raccoon joins the scene. In an almost comedic fashion, the raccoon poses here long enough for a camera to be brought to this site and photographed.

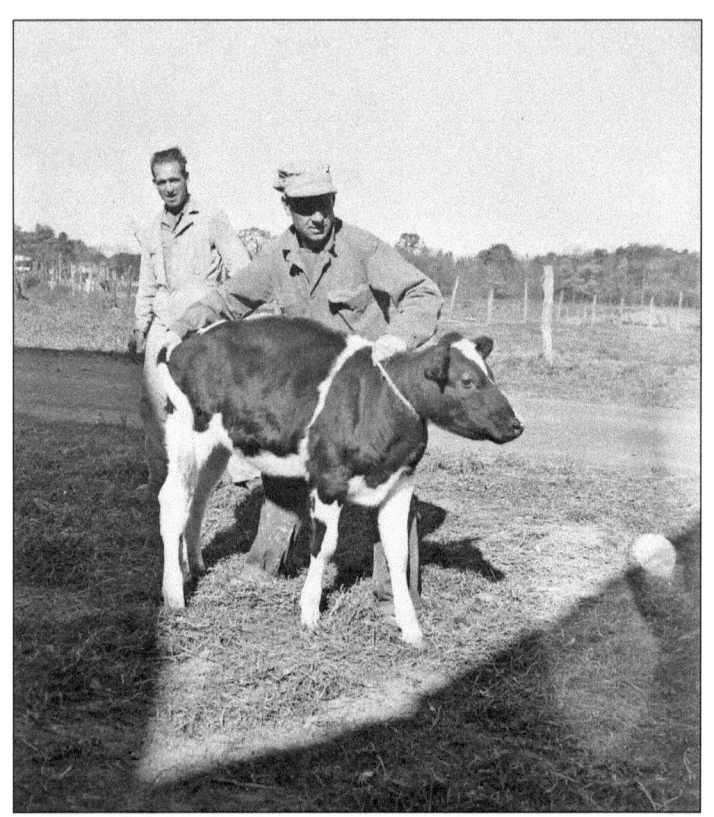

Dairy cows were a familiar sight on the hospital farm. At left is a calf at the newly constructed dairy barn a few years into its operation in the early 20th century. Below is an inside look into the milking parlor of the dairy barn. One milkman can be seen moving about the building with stainless steel pails used for collecting milk by hand. This was a place where paid farmers and patients worked together to accomplish the necessary work of providing food for the hospital kitchen. Feeding, herding, and milking enough cows to supply hundreds of people with milk for daily use was no small charge.

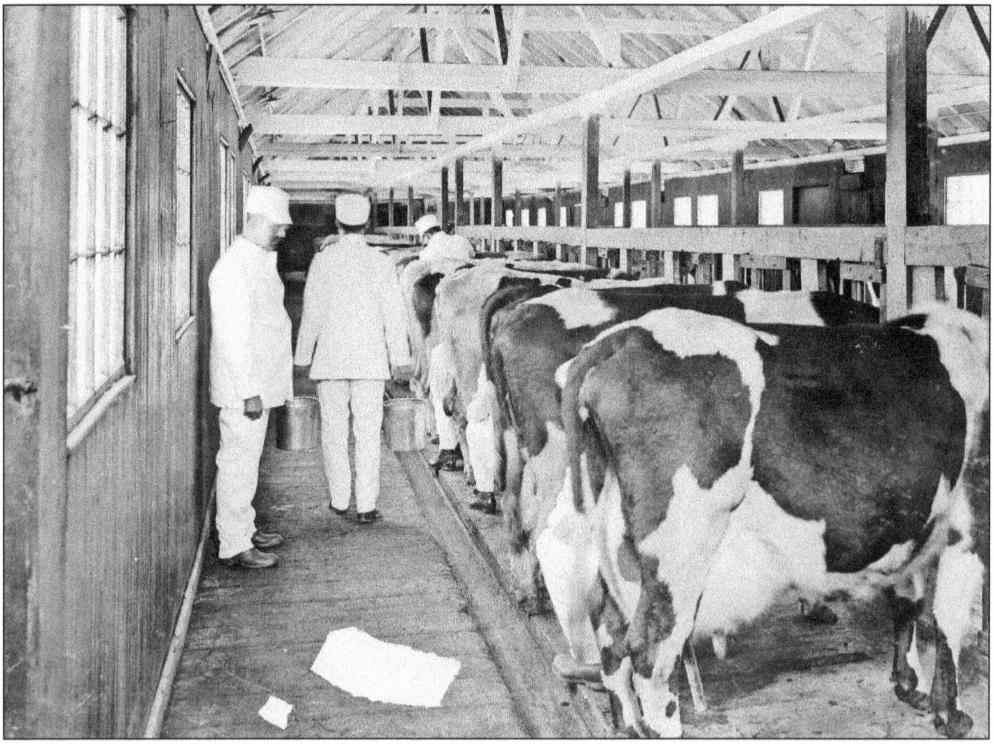

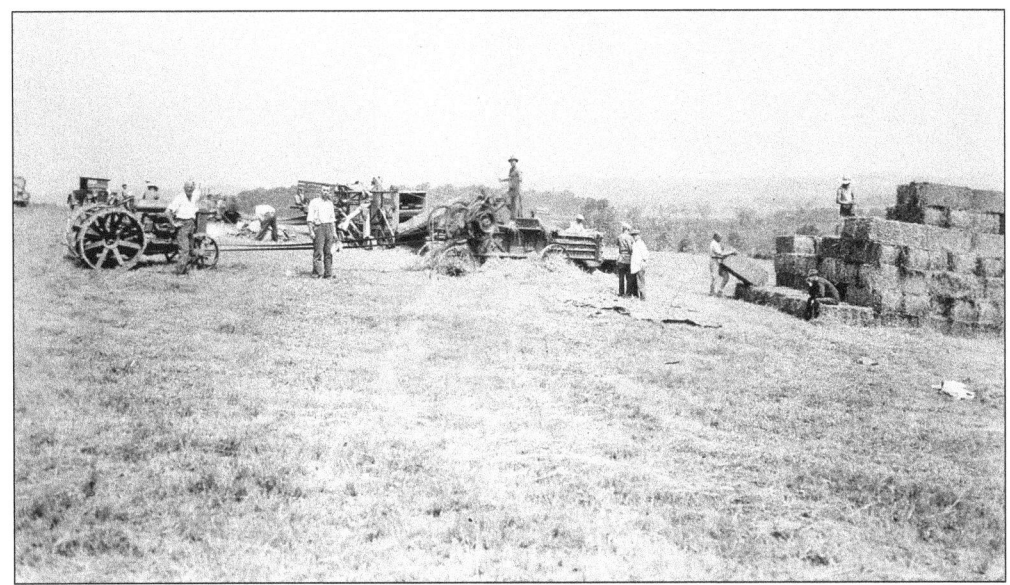

Hay was a staple of all barns with animals, as it was used for bedding. It also served a critical role in controlling soil erosion and helped keep weeds down in fields. The 1920s image shows farmers and likely patient workers teaming up to collect hay. It was then piled onto trucks and flats for transport.

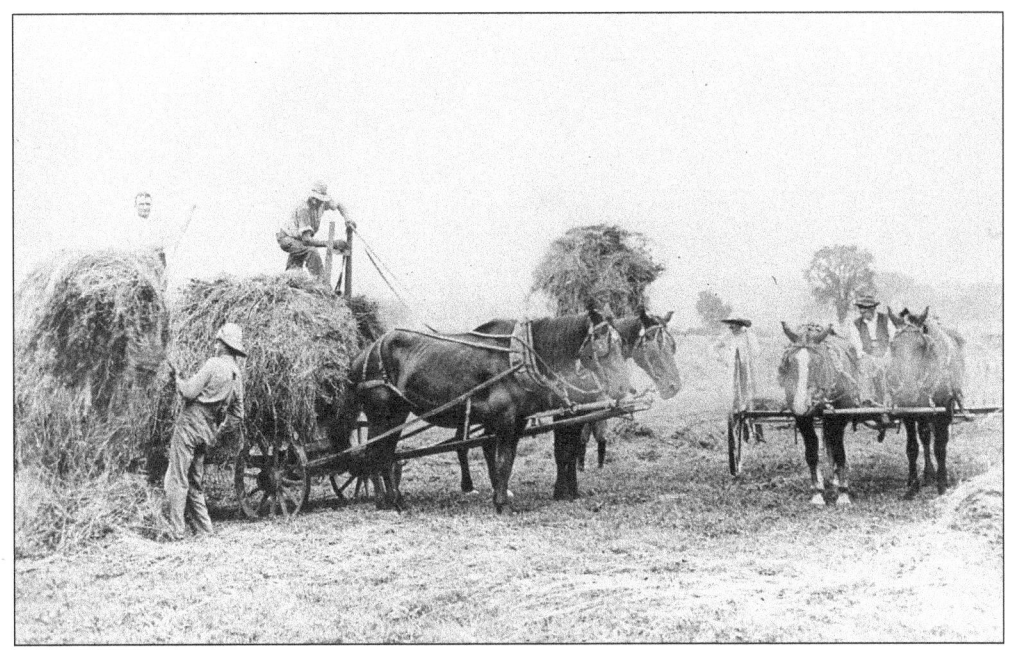

Before the advent of automobiles and mechanized farm equipment, gathering hay for the hospital was even more labor intensive. This 19th-century image shows men using rakes and pitchforks to gather hay into large piles. Aside from use on the farm, hay was used in the shops as stuffing for early mattresses and cushions.

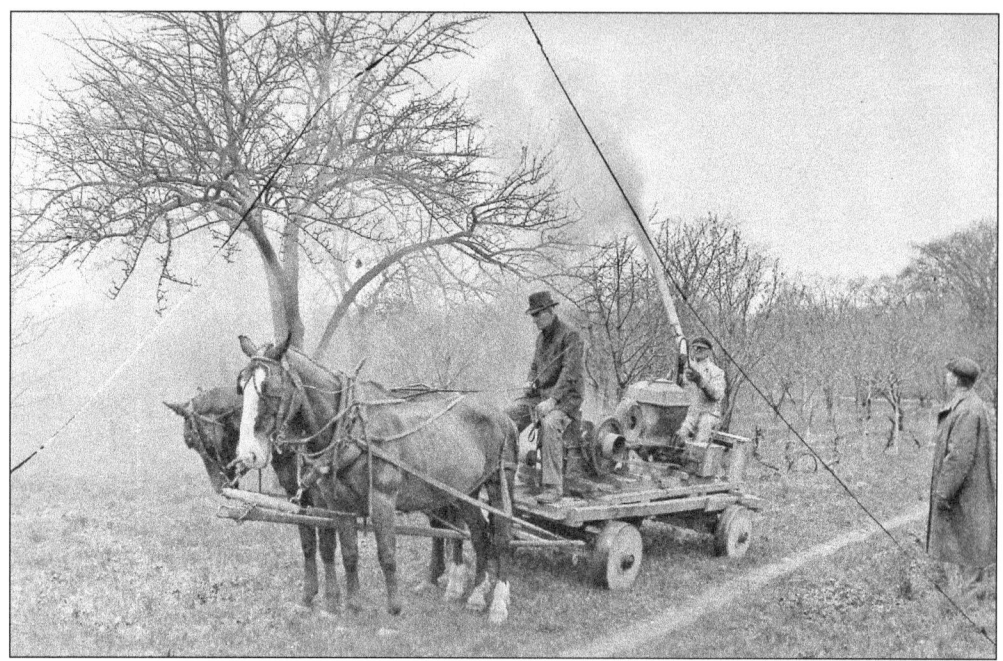

Aside from livery and annual crops, maintaining trees and shrubs was a duty of farm staff. Here, men spray fruit trees with fertilizer. Apples could be found in large groves on the hospital grounds. As a by-product of yearly trimmings, applewood was then used for smoking meats at the facility.

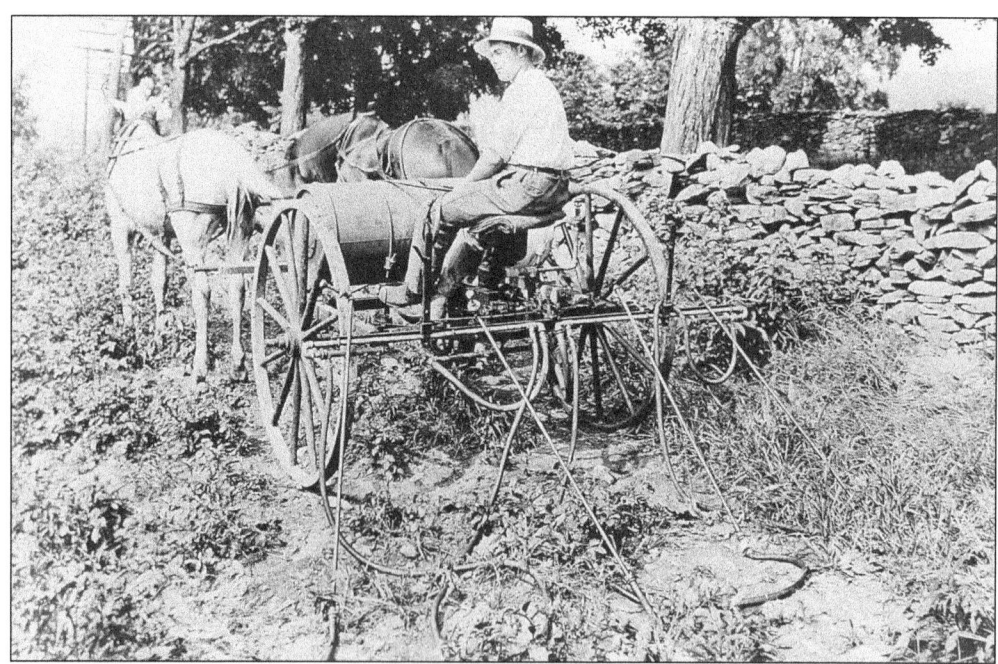

Before modern sprinkler systems, the hospital farmland operated on a system of sloped drainage through the fields from rain. In times of drought, crops would need manual watering. Here a farmhand uses a horse-drawn system to irrigate peas in the spring. Hoses attached to a tank were dragged behind and fed water by gravity.

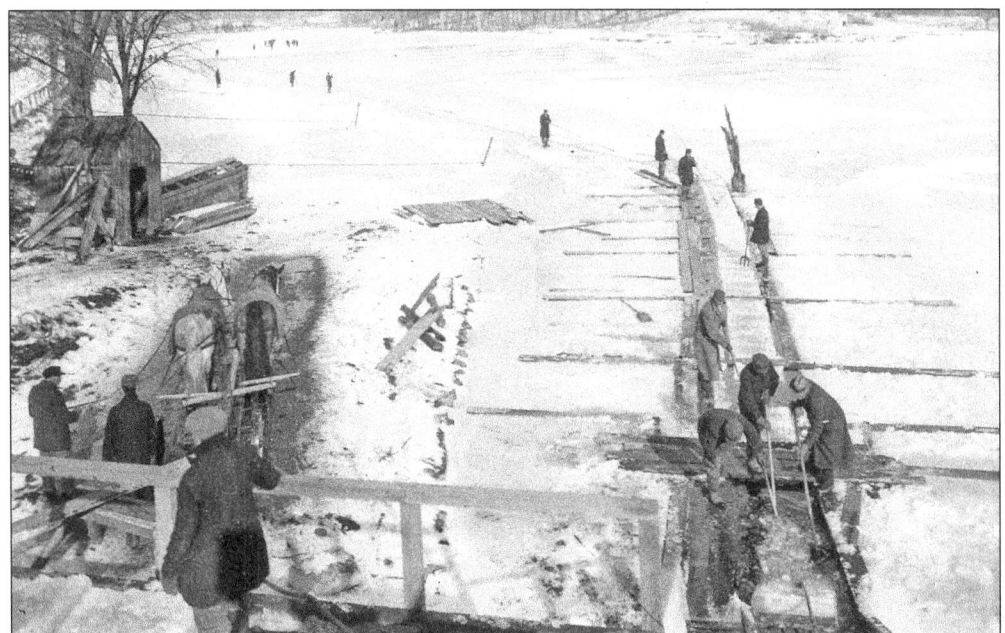

Ice cut from nearby Fall Kill Creek was a means of cooling utilized until modern refrigeration was invented. Here a crew of men can be seen using simple equipment to remove blocks of ice from the creek's surface. Ice was carted back to the hospital via a horse and carriage.

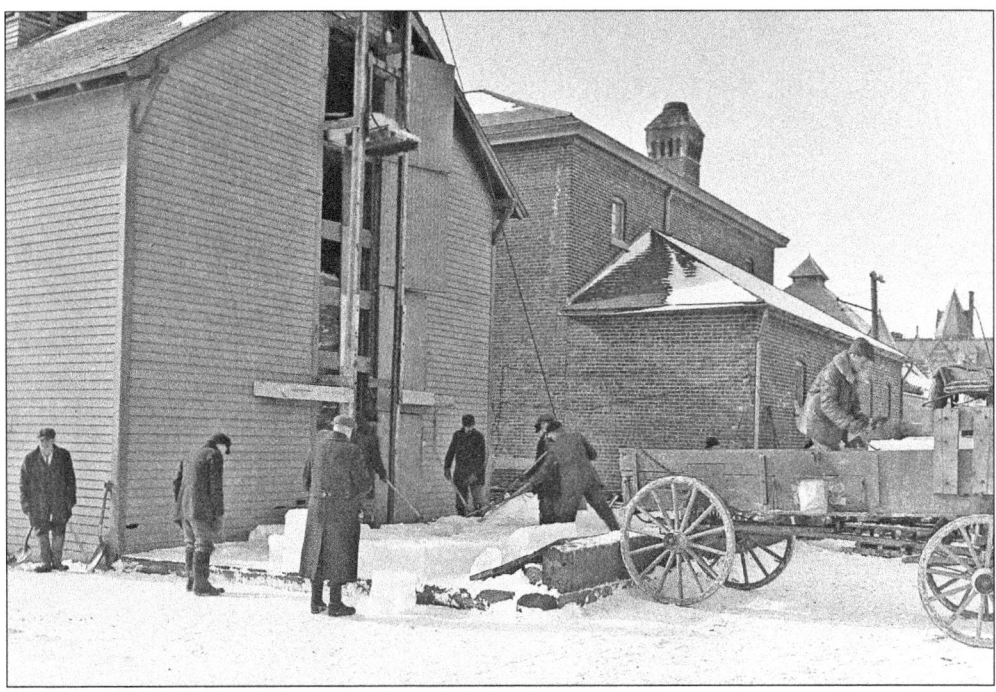

Just behind the old storehouse sat the wooden icehouse shown here. Ice harvested from the creek was brought here for storage and central distribution. A rope and pulley moved the ice off the concrete platform up into a loft. This image was taken around the turn of the century.

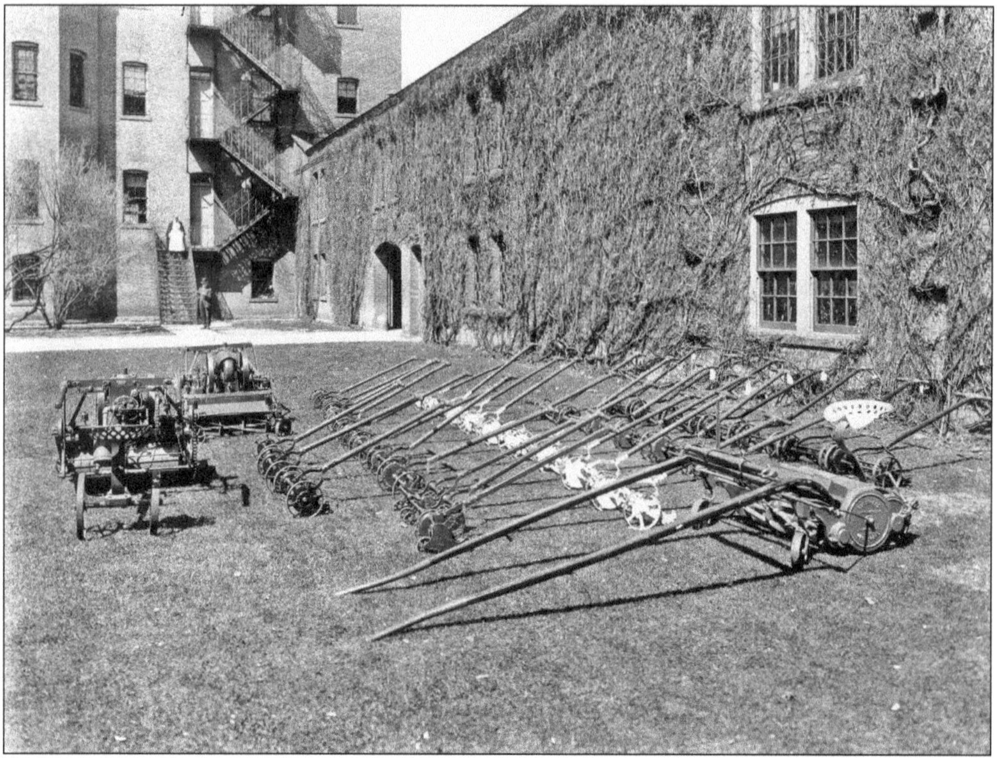

Aside from patient work squads who maintained the grounds, farm staff also acted as groundskeepers. This image shows the manual mowers that would have cut the hospital fields. The early riding lawn mower to the front right was horse powered. In the background, a nurse exits the main building on the metal stairs.

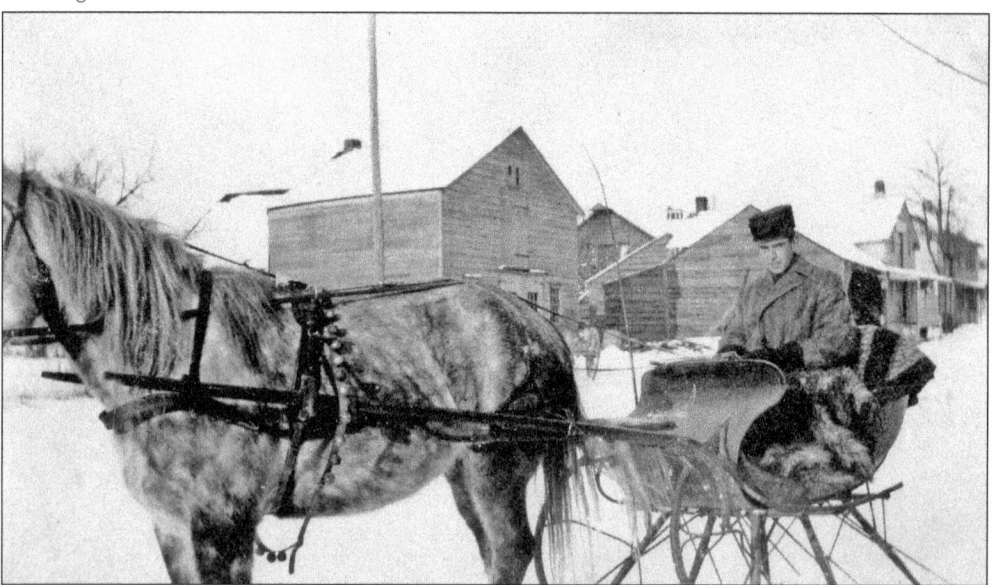

Horse Nelly pulls a sled near the farm. In the background sits a few loosely constructed wooden buildings. Some served as barns, and some were shanties built of scrap lumber. These shanty buildings were makeshift places for farmers to stay out of the elements.

Six

PATIENT LIFE AND ACTIVITIES

In order to have a scheduled day plan for patients to adapt and follow, a ward routine was established. Patients were awoken around 6:00 to 6:30 a.m. Breakfast was served in the dining halls between 7:00 and 8:00 a.m., and patients had to be washed and dressed before then. At the end of each meal, all silverware was counted by staff. If anything was missing, no patients could leave the dining hall until it was located. This was not only for the risk of a weapon but also because crafty individuals could shape silverware to be used in an escape. After returning to the ward from breakfast, those patients who had a vocation at the hospital went off to their respective work squads. Those who remained on the ward would assist in chores on the unit if willing and able. Housework such as collecting laundry, making beds, and polishing floors were common patient jobs. Lunch was served promptly at noon and dinner at six in the evening. Lights out was around nine at night for patients. Barbers came three times per week to shave men and cut hair. Beauticians were made available to female patients as well.

Wednesday and Sunday were visiting days, and religious services were also on Sunday for Catholics and Protestants. Saturday was for Jewish services and seasonal sports. Monday was a time where male and female patients mixed in dance events at the Assembly Hall. Tuesday and Friday were for physical activity, walking, and recreation. Thursday was movie night. Work and activity engagement were a part of treatment, and the subsequent labor meant the hospital was able to self-produce necessities ranging from machine parts to shoes. Work was never forced, but it was rewarded and encouraged. Profession largely is how individuals define a part of their personhood and is an extremely valued part of life for all. Allowing psychiatric patients to continue their trade while hospitalized was undoubtedly a dignified act. Additionally, crafting amenities such as soap, clothing, and reeds for basketmaking were all part of facilitating a self-sufficient hospital community.

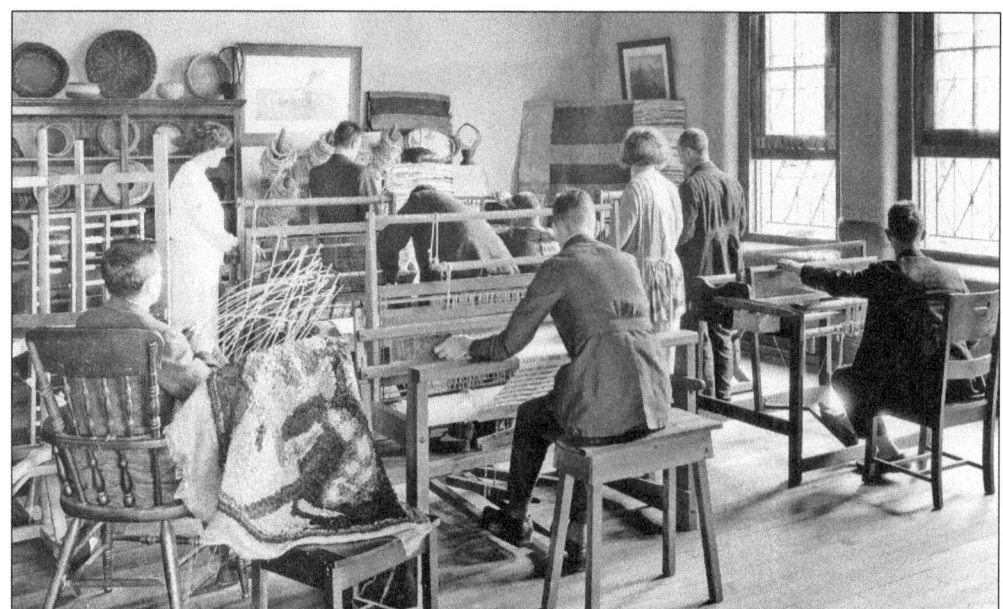

Occupational therapy was the core of patient activities until after World War II. After the war, occupational therapy split into two separate entities, recreation therapy and traditional vocational related activity, which remained under the guise of occupational therapy. Basket weaving was a popular activity for male patients. This 1921 image shows men in the main building weaving baskets and mats.

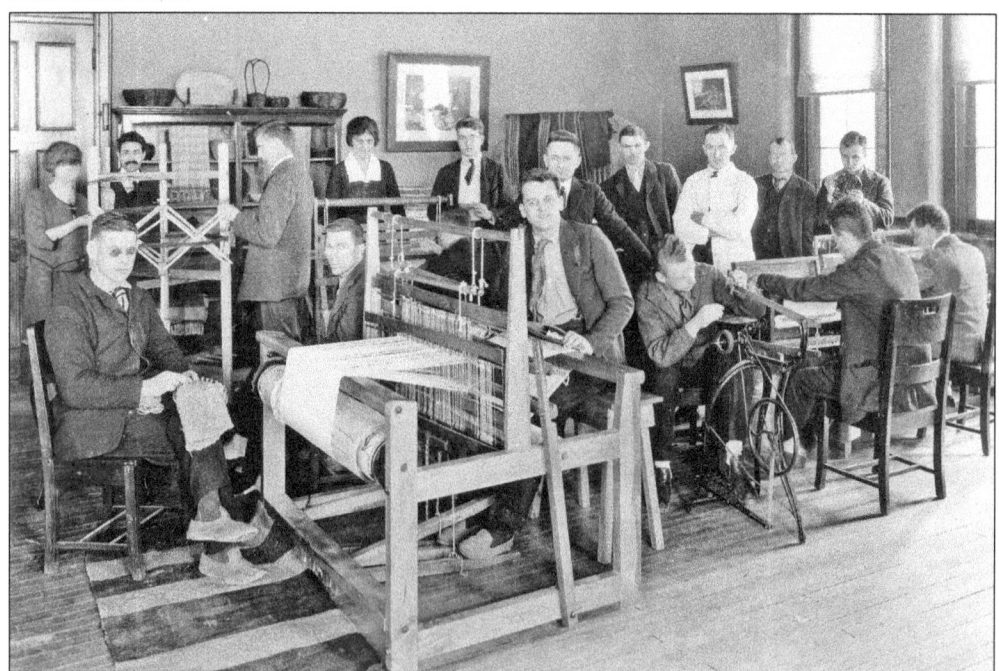

This tailor shop in the main building was run by men. Here finishing touches were applied to clothing or articles in need of fitting. Woven sheets, cloths, and other material articles were also produced. Notice the appearance of the men, all in clothing and shoes fitted perfectly to each individual.

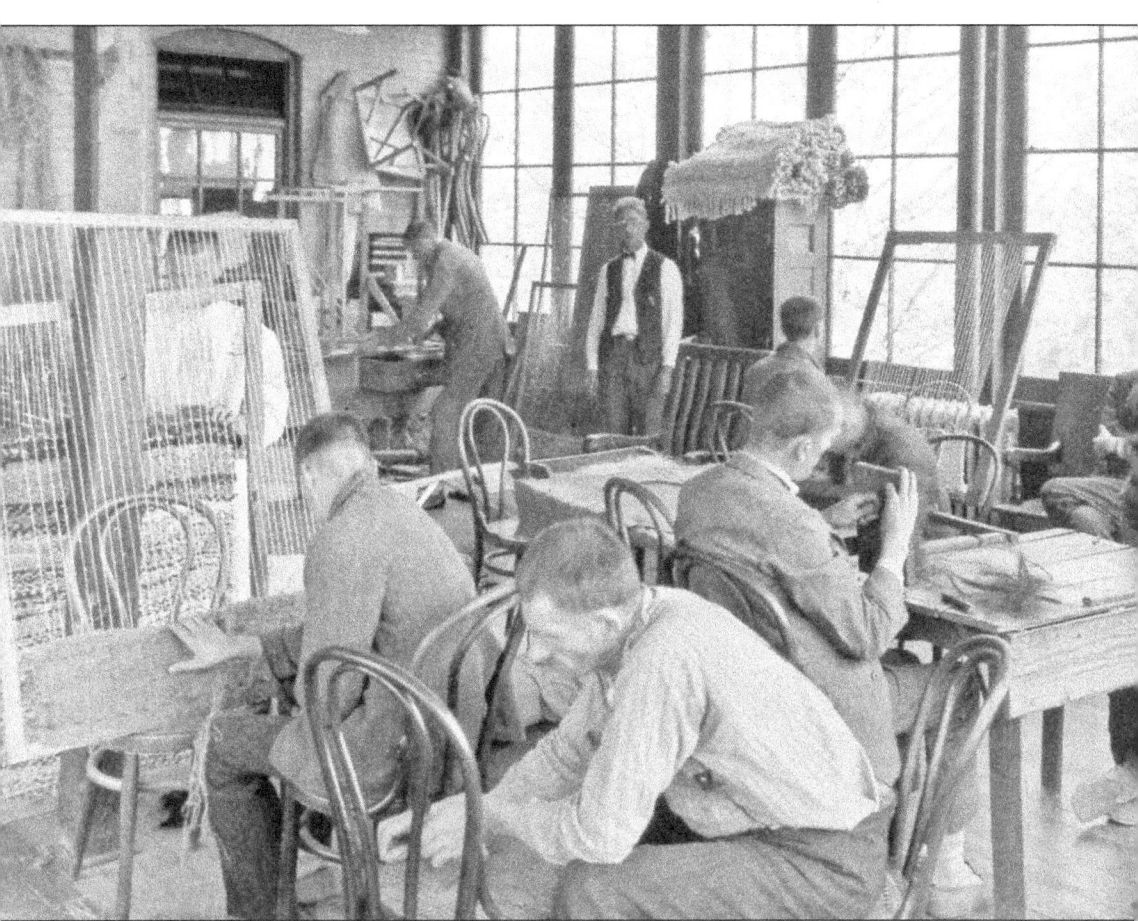

As space became limited with a growing population, areas were repurposed to accommodate rooms for occupational therapy. This image was taken in a porch in the Central Group converted to an occupational therapy workshop. On the floor to the right, scraps of cloth are recycled to make a woven rug. In the center, a male is working on caning the seat of a chair. No material was wasted in these times. Caning chairs and basket weaving tended to be more male-dominated activity at Hudson River State Hospital, while weaving and sewing were generally more female-dominated. Both sexes did engage in these activates if they wished. Without electronic entertainment in this time, these were considered leisure activities and greatly enjoyed by the many who wished to participate.

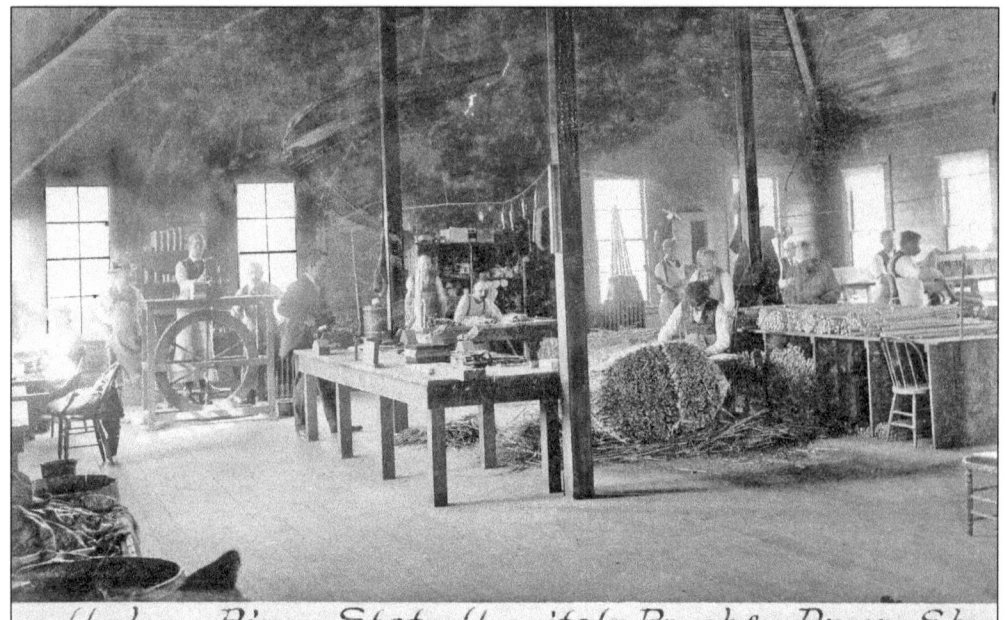

Very few everyday articles were not produced at the hospital in earlier times. This early-20th-century image was taken in the broom shop. To the right on a table sit wooden handles. On the floor sits a pile of sturdy straw for use as the sweep mechanism of the broom.

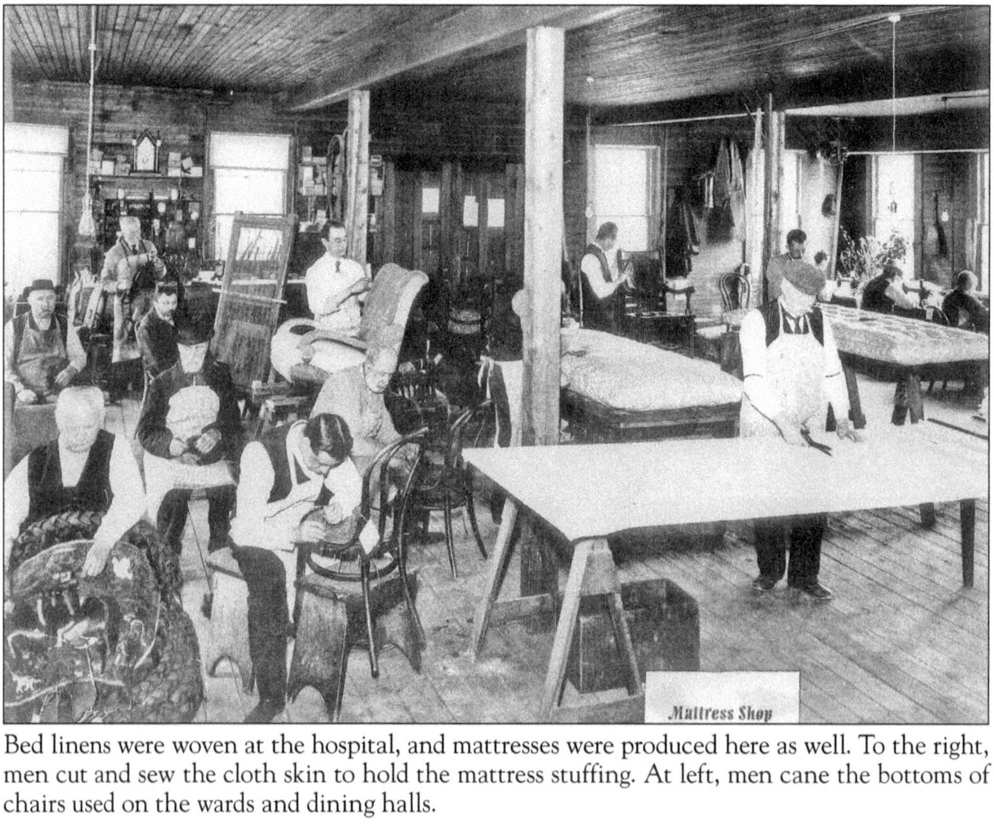

Bed linens were woven at the hospital, and mattresses were produced here as well. To the right, men cut and sew the cloth skin to hold the mattress stuffing. At left, men cane the bottoms of chairs used on the wards and dining halls.

Trade amongst state facilities was a feature of the state system in the 19th and early 20th centuries. This 1904 order for women's shoes was from another state institution at Kings Park on Long Island. Notice no actual cash cost was due, rather the debt is placed in a fund. When the supplying hospital was in need of a good, it would use this credit to purchase said good from Hudson River.

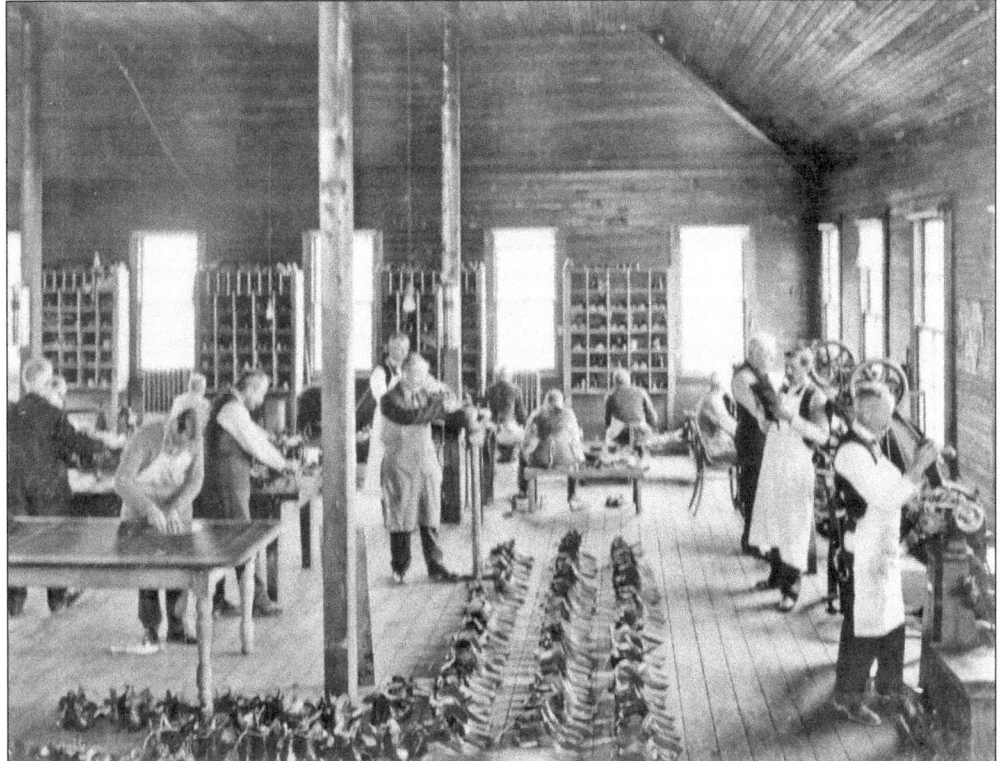

It is hard to argue that shoes are not an important item of dress. In the early 20th century, men work to cobble shoes for the hospital. Just as in society, shoemaking was generally a male-dominated job at Hudson River. In the center sit dozens of completed shoes.

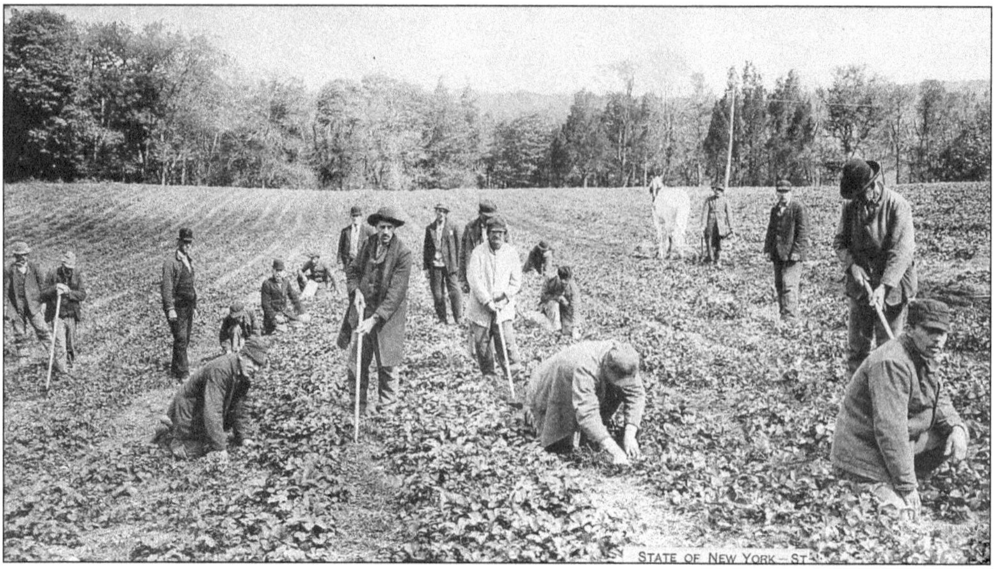

Aside from working in shops, aiding on the grounds of the hospital was an activity that many men assisted with. Duties could range from cutting grass and planting crops to harvesting. Here, men assist in weeding the rows of crops planted at the hospital farm.

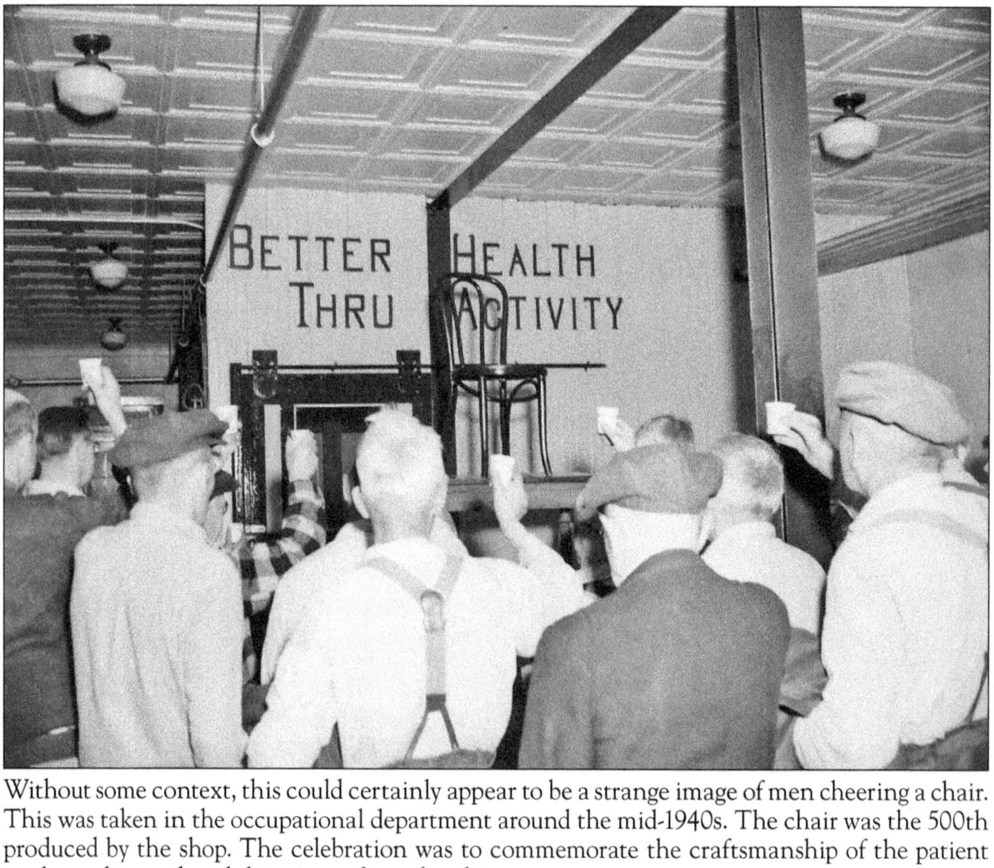

Without some context, this could certainly appear to be a strange image of men cheering a chair. This was taken in the occupational department around the mid-1940s. The chair was the 500th produced by the shop. The celebration was to commemorate the craftsmanship of the patient workers who produced this piece of woodworking.

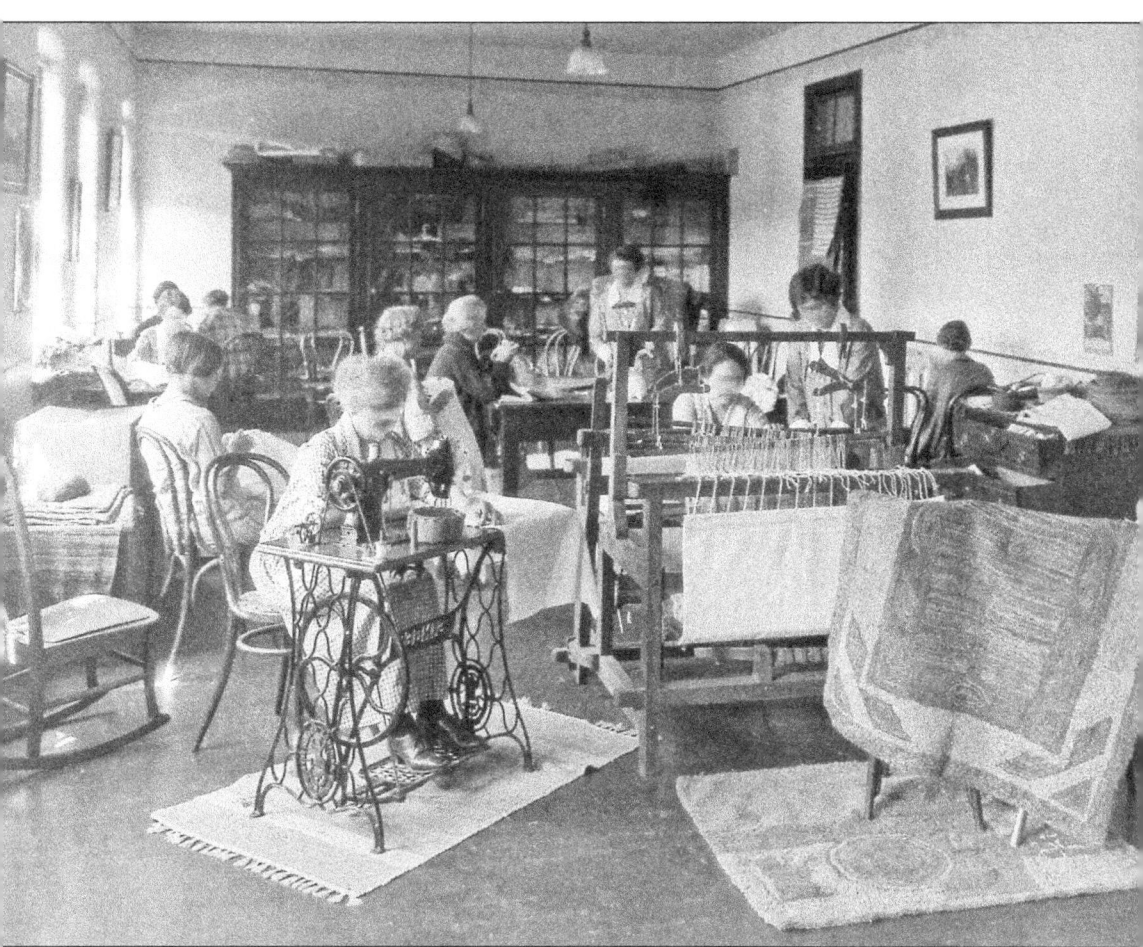

For female patients, sewing and looming were commonplace activities at Hudson River, as they were in broad society at the time. This 1910s image shows an occupational therapy room in the main building's north wing. Note that the sewing machine in front is foot-powered, not electric. Two completed rugs sit on display. Skillfully crafted items such as these were often put on display at hospital occupational therapy exhibits. This gave others in the hospital the opportunity to see the talent of so many of the individuals who resided at Hudson River for themselves. Items were available for sale at some of these exhibits or in the occupational therapy store. Whenever goods were sold, with the patient's permission, the patient earned a portion of the sale's proceeds in cash or tokens to spend at the community store.

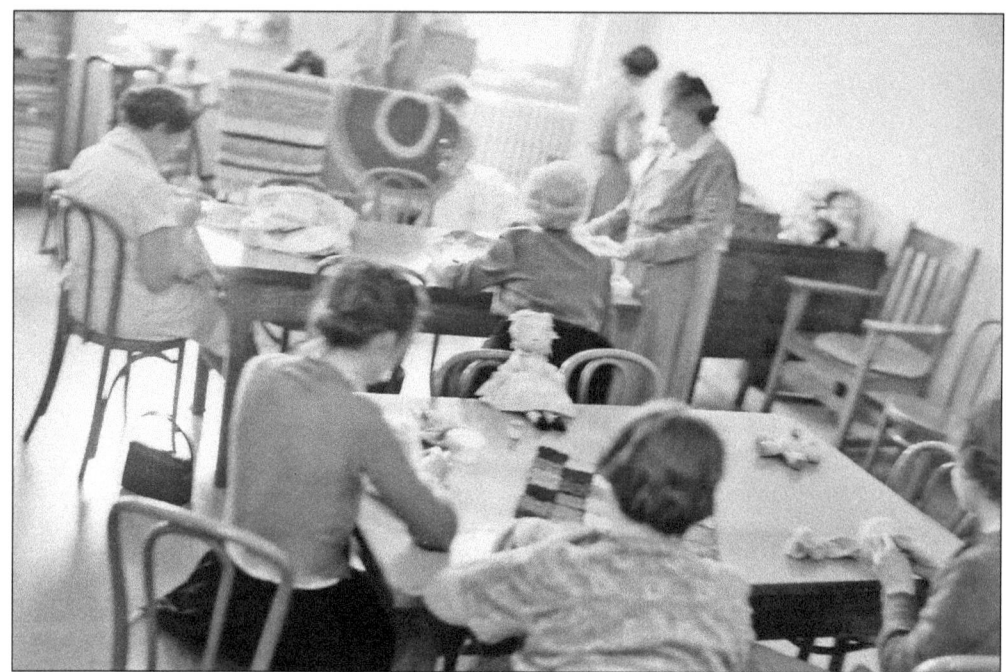

Not all patients were able to leave their building or ward to go out into separate, and sometimes far, shop buildings because of walking ability. This photograph, taken in Ryon Hall in 1951, shows an occupational therapy class for such patients. Here a group of older women makes children's toys.

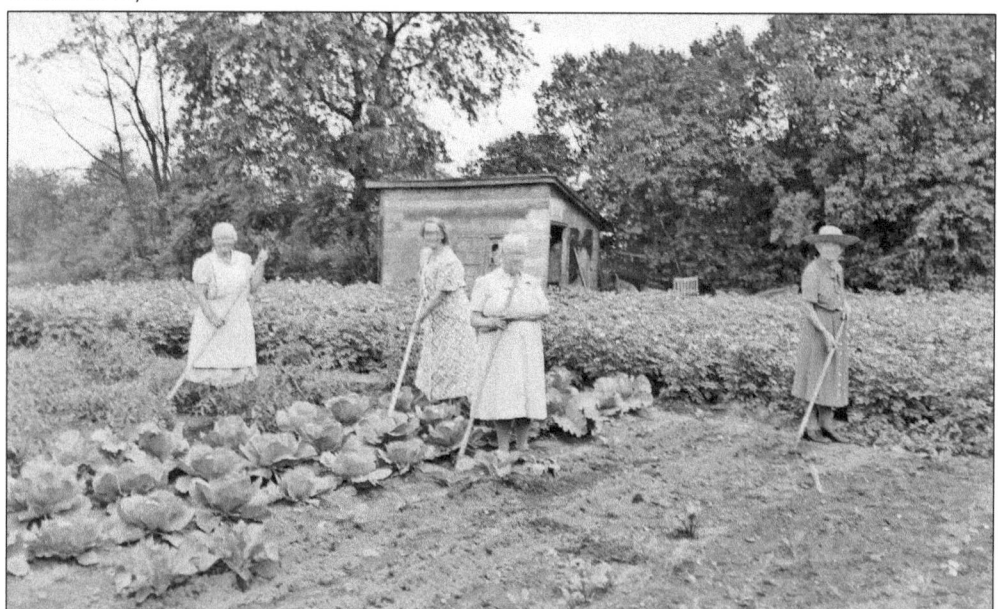

When it came to supporting the operations of the farm, there were jobs to be had for all who were interested. This early-spring photograph taken in the 1940s shows women tending crops grown from seeds in the greenhouse. This was more than just about vegetable production, this was about making the patients at Hudson River feel that they were valued and had purpose through vocation as the rest of society does.

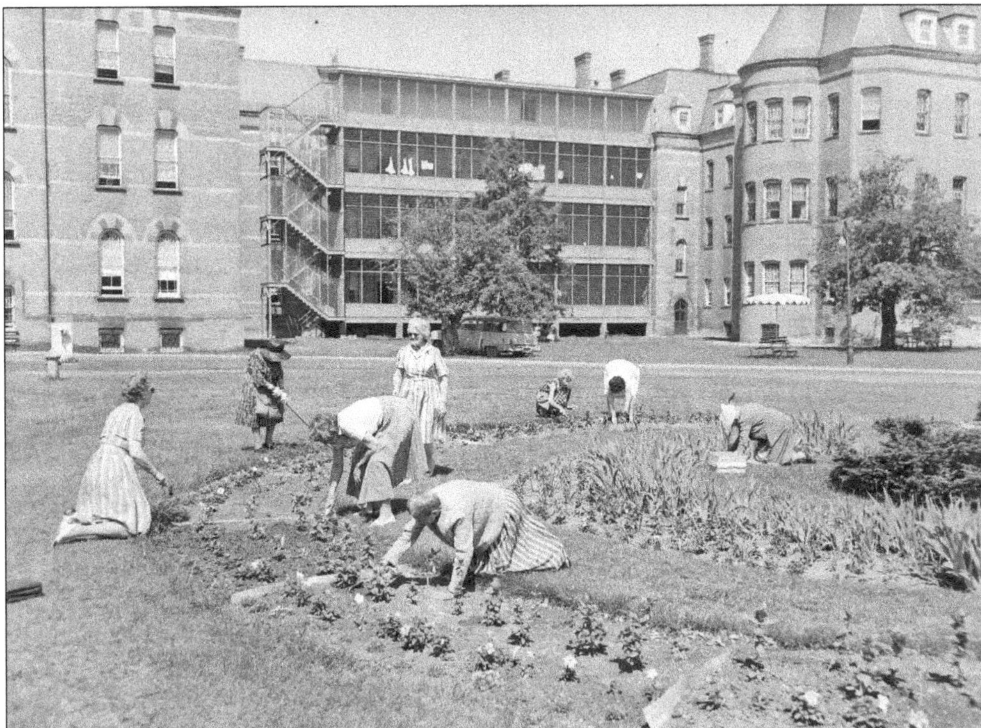

Ornamental gardening was a common feature of the neatly manicured grounds at Hudson River. Often individual groups or wards were given small plots of land for a flower garden to call their own. Here women tend to a circular garden behind the north wing of the main building.

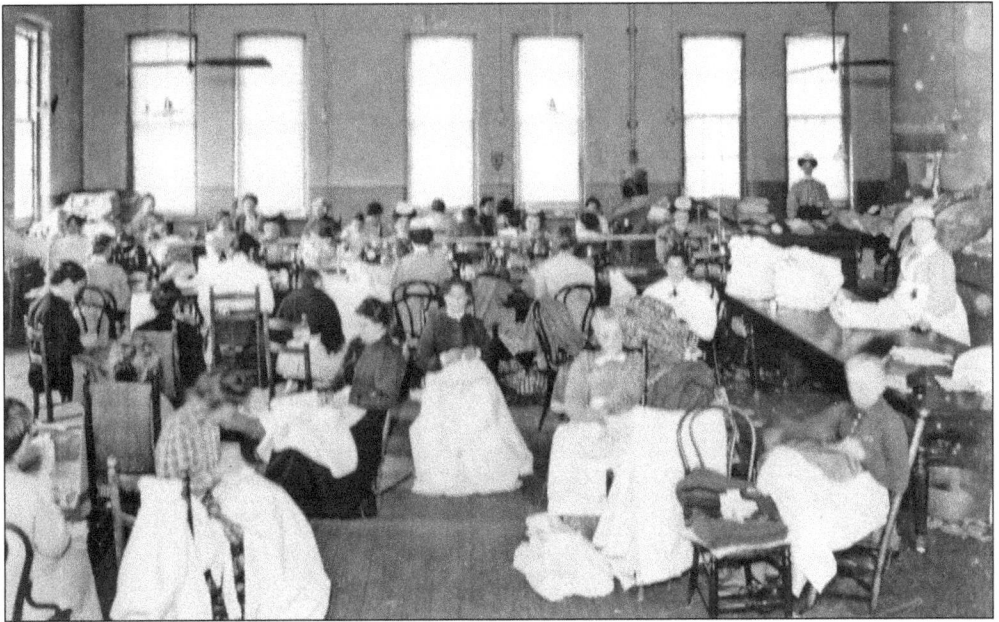

This early-20th-century image was taken in the hospital laundry. Women work together to mend tears in linens. At right, a nurse stands by the folding table. The blue-and-white uniform with a massive wad of keys can be immediately spotted.

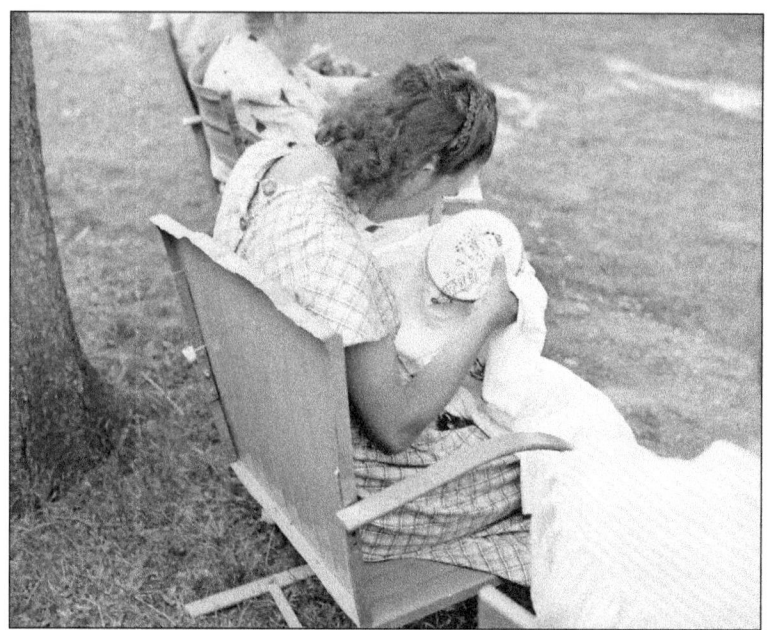

Contrary to public opinion, the majority of patients at the hospital spent little time locked up on the wards. Whenever weather permitted, patients spent time on the grounds in secured or unsecured areas dependent on privilege level. Here, a group of women partake in the leisure activity of needlepoint on a spring day.

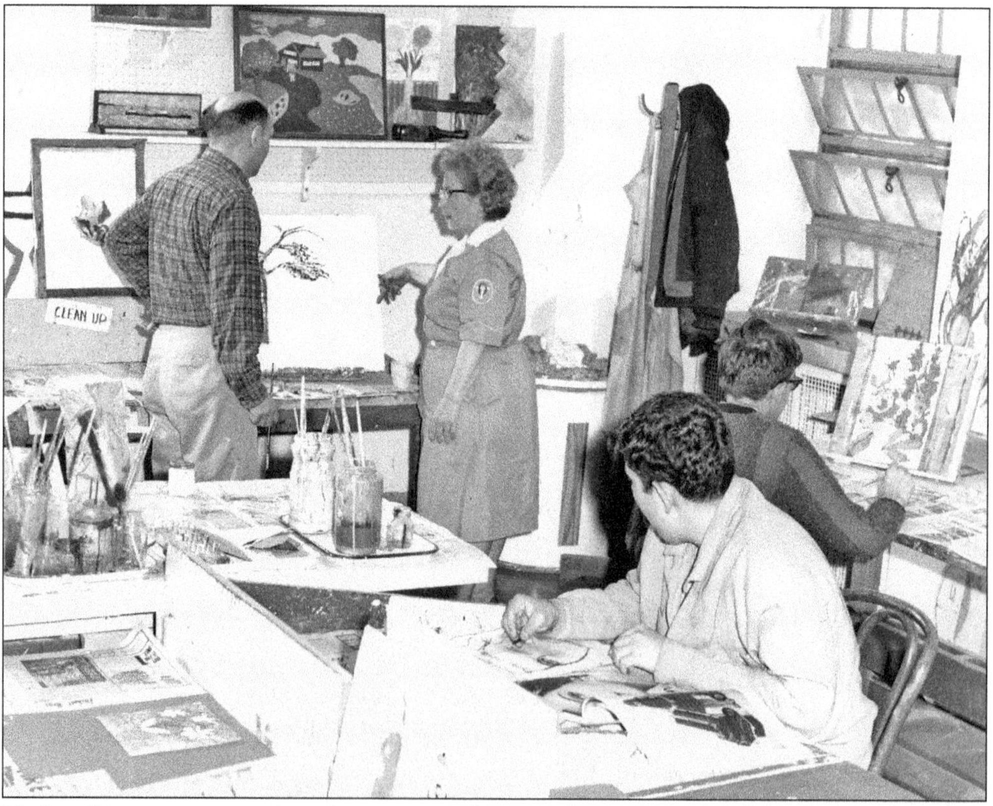

Hudson River saw some talented artists over the years. Regardless of skill level, individuals who were interested in paint or art were encouraged to express their creativity. Here, an occupational therapy aid instructs an individual how to paint on canvas. In the background sits complete artwork as an encouragement to those less skilled to develop their talent.

As technology advanced and new jobs emerged, programs at the hospital developed to acclimate according to the time. This image taken in the 1960s in Cheney Memorial shows one such class. Individuals are taught to operate IBM's newly invented technology by occupational therapy instructors.

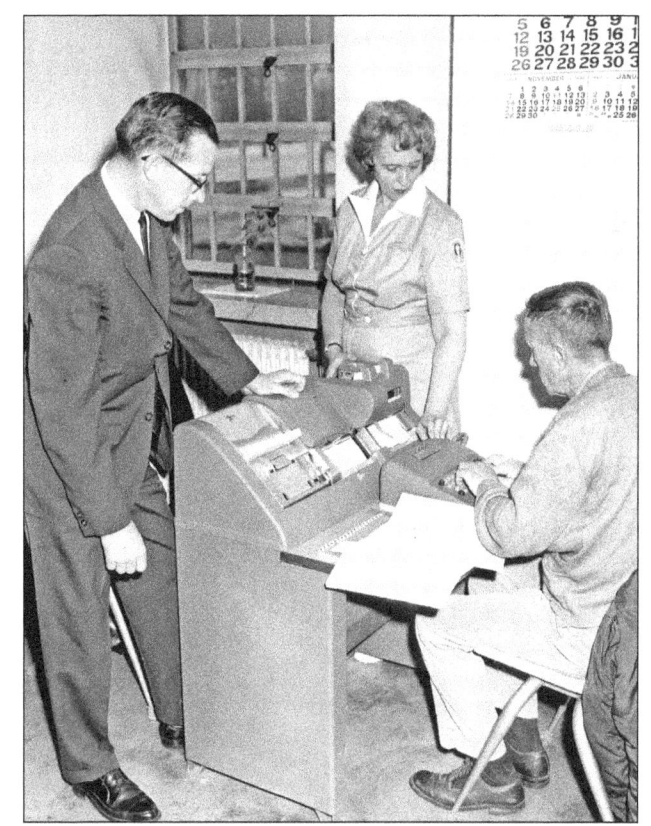

This turn-of-the-century image shows the Assembly Hall in the main building before a separate building was constructed. Here, articles made in the various shops and occupational therapy departments all over the hospital were on display and for sale. Patients received a portion of the proceeds if items they crafted were sold.

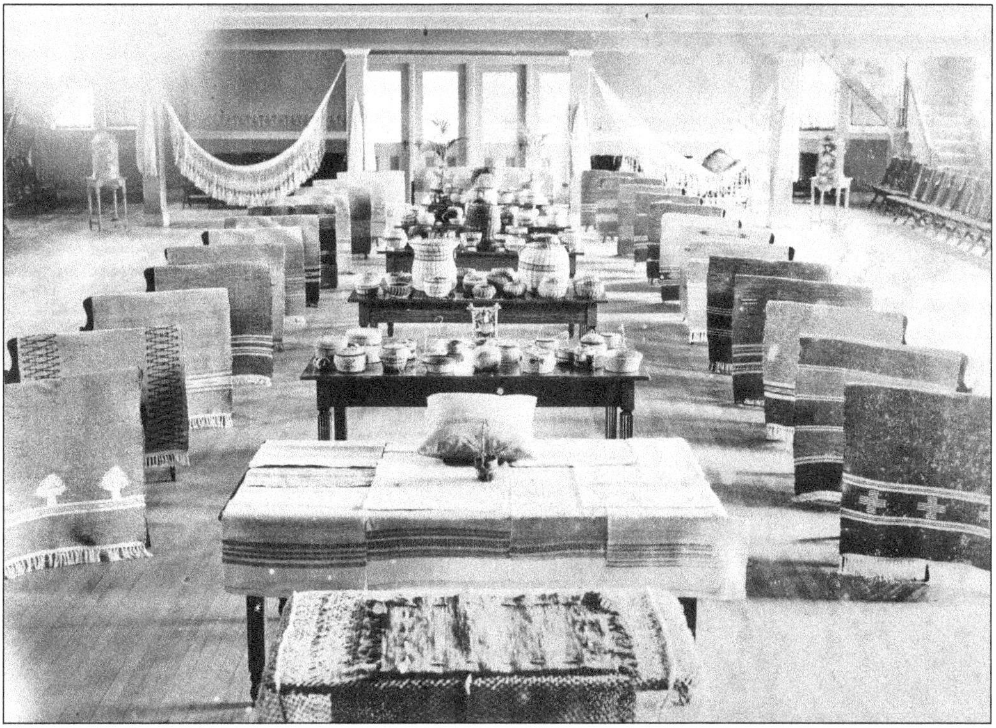

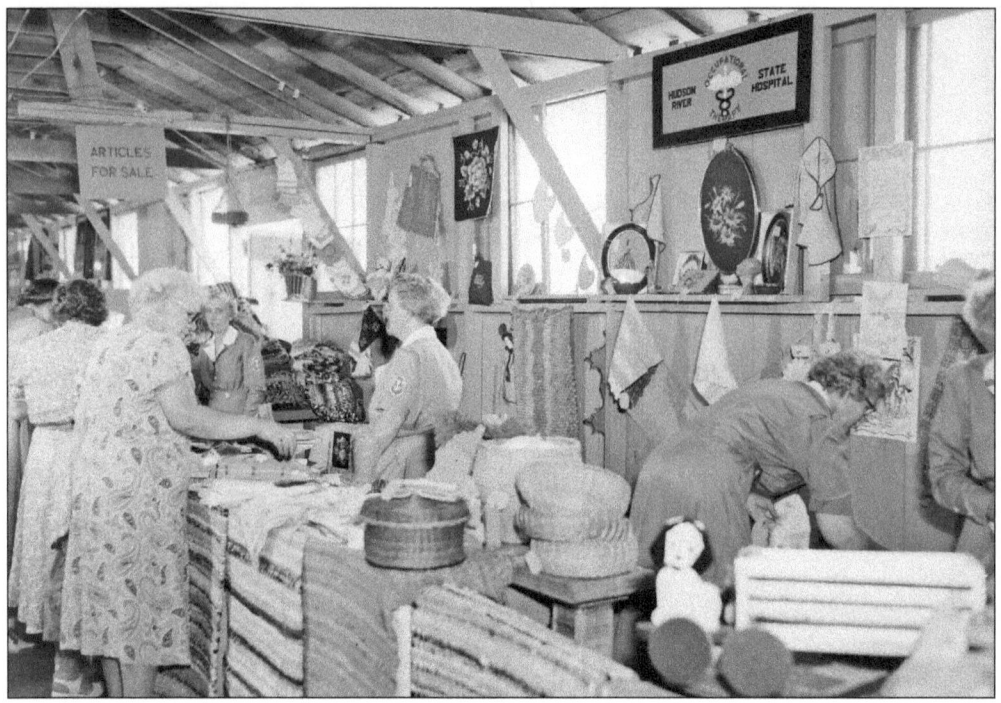

Another popular place to sell articles made at the hospital was the Dutchess County Fair. This image taken in August 1952 showcases an exhibit from the hospital. Items from baskets to rugs to farm produce were displayed proudly. This was an opportunity to show off publicly the talent of so many creative and industrious individuals at Hudson River.

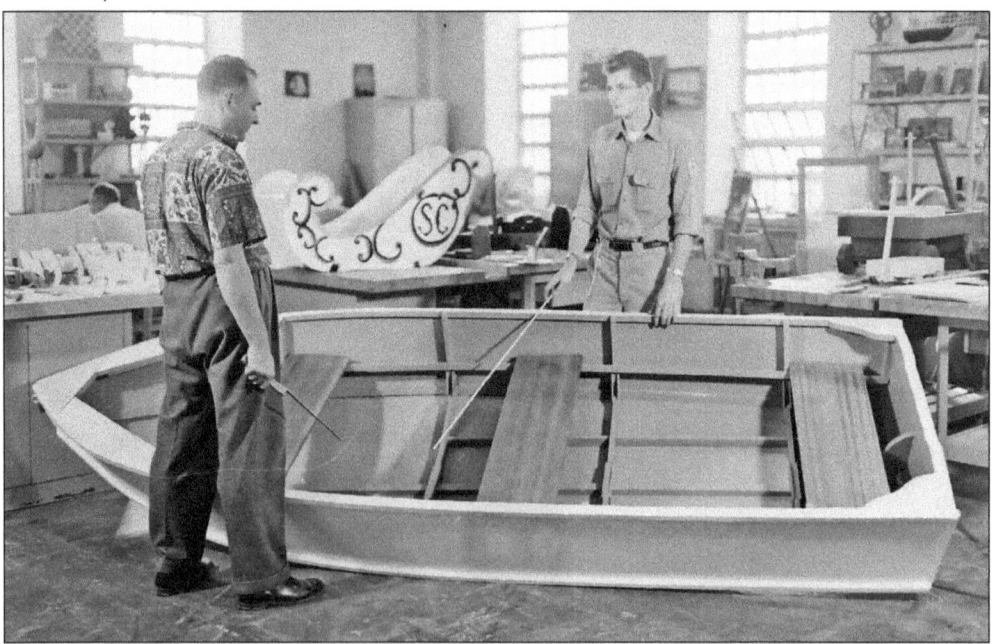

Some very talented individuals lived and worked at Hudson River. Here, a boat is skillfully crafted from wood. On a table to the rear sits a wonderfully ornate Christmas sled. Items like this would often be put on display in common areas of the building for all to enjoy.

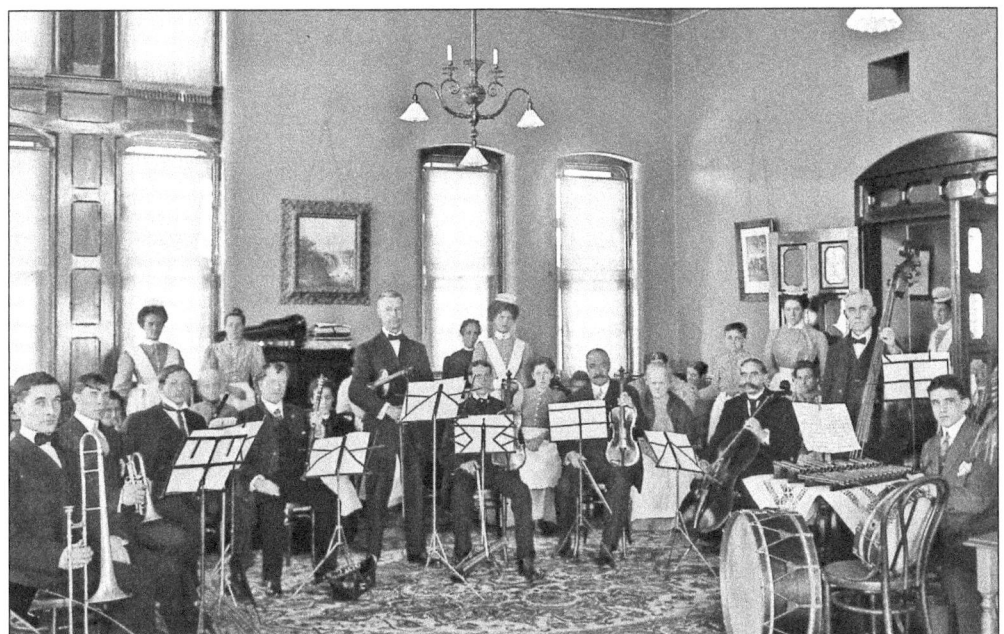

Music was encouraged at the hospital from the earliest days. Here, the hospital band practices a number in the main building. The band would play in events on the grounds and in the many plays produced by patients in the hospital. In later years, research would prove that music, dance, and cooperative activity are some of the most beneficial cognitive exercise for individuals.

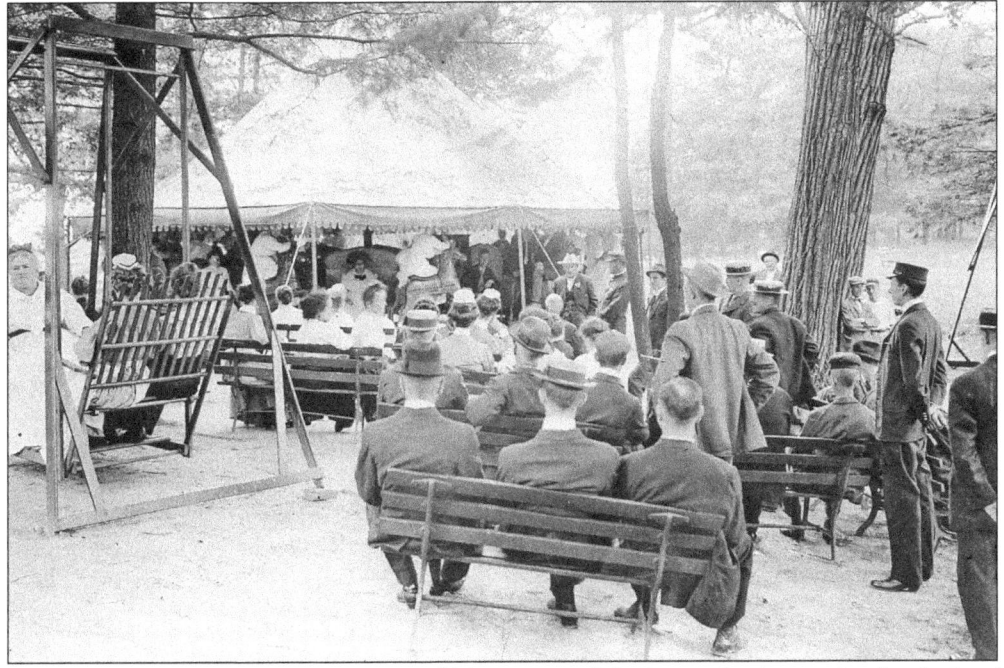

Spring was a time for all to enjoy the parklike setting of the hospital, often under the shade of towering pines. This spring social event shows a carousel under the tent for staff and patients to enjoy. This is a fine image to dispel the common misconception that all patients spent most their time on locked wards.

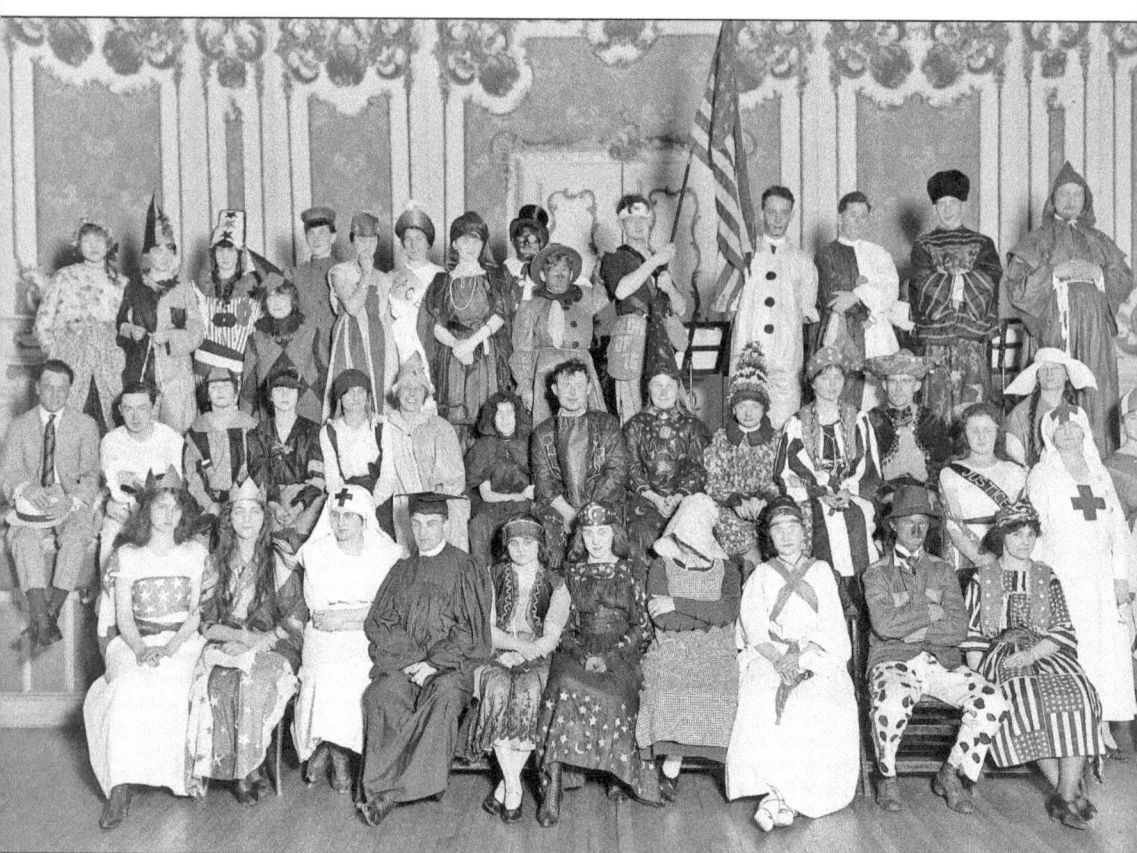

In the early days, the Assembly Hall was one of the few places patients of opposite sex would mingle socially. The first Assembly Hall was in the north wing of the main building until a separate, free-standing building was constructed. This 1918 image in the main building Assembly Hall shows the cast of a masquerade ball. These types of shows were held several times per year at Hudson River, sometimes outdoors weather permitting in warmer parts of the year. These events often began with a play onstage telling a specific story, followed by a dance event in costume for all to enjoy. Costumes were made by patients with the help of occupational therapy staff in groups according to the genre of the masquerade.

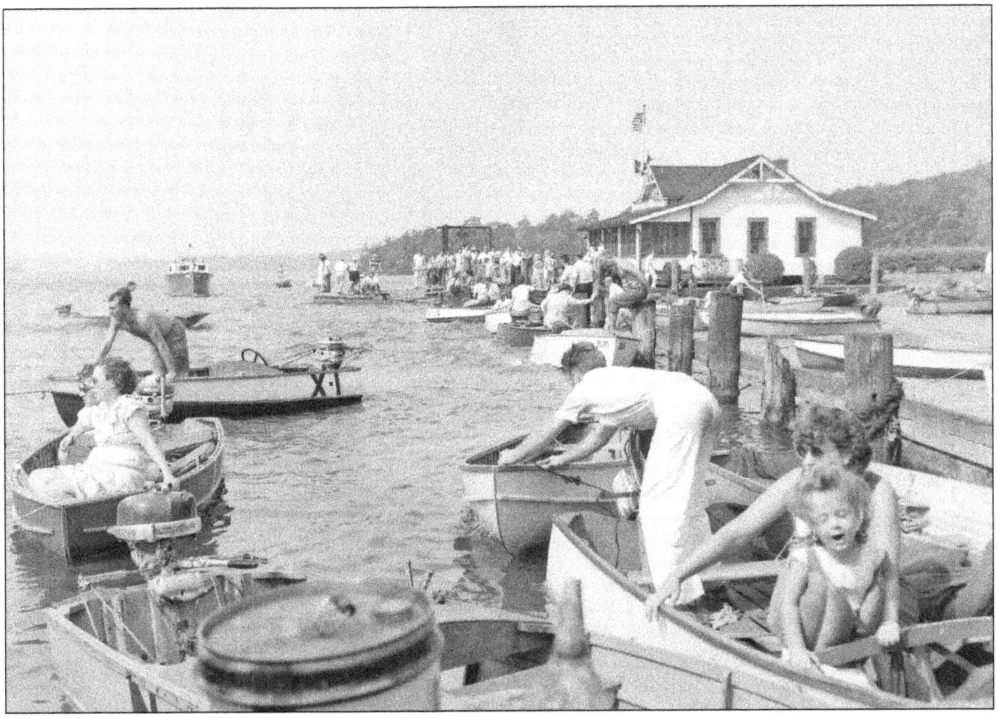

As well as providing a scenic view all year long, the Hudson River provided many recreational opportunities for staff and patients. This 1950s scene shows people of all ages enjoying a group outing down the river. Fishing was also a source of great fun for many.

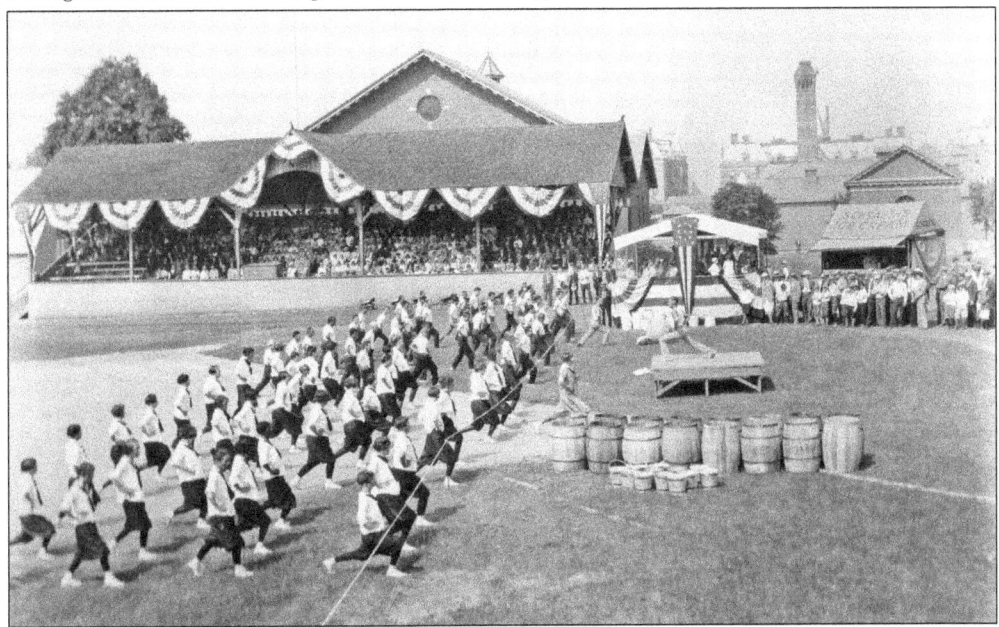

This 1920s image shows a patriotic summer field day. Women on the drill team at center display cooperative movement techniques learned during the year. This was an excellent source of physical activity that engaged cognitive function as well. In front of the group stands the drill leader modeling moves.

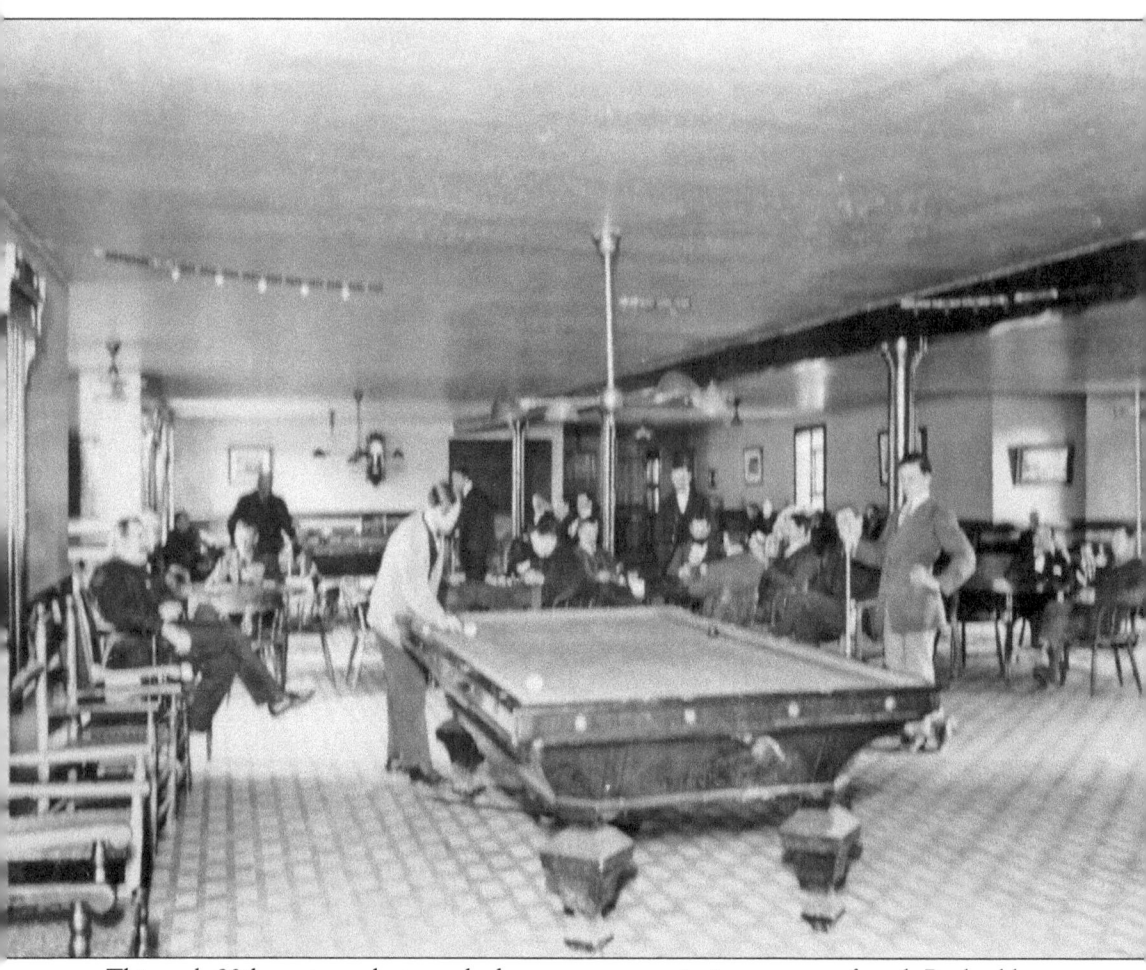

This early-20th-century photograph showcases men enjoying a game of pool. Pool tables were common to most male wards and employee social areas. This is an example of an area at the hospital where the mingling of male and female staff would be considered "fraternizing" on duty and therefore inappropriate. This area was shared by staff and patients for recreational activity. In the background, other gentlemen are gathered around card games. Take notice of the sharp dress of the men, a familiar sight in this era of Hudson River. Since most of the clothes were made in the hospital tailor shop when this image was taken, personal measurements were taken and clothes fitted for patients. This gave them the same dignity as any other man or woman of the day in everyday society and sometimes better dress than they could afford on the outside.

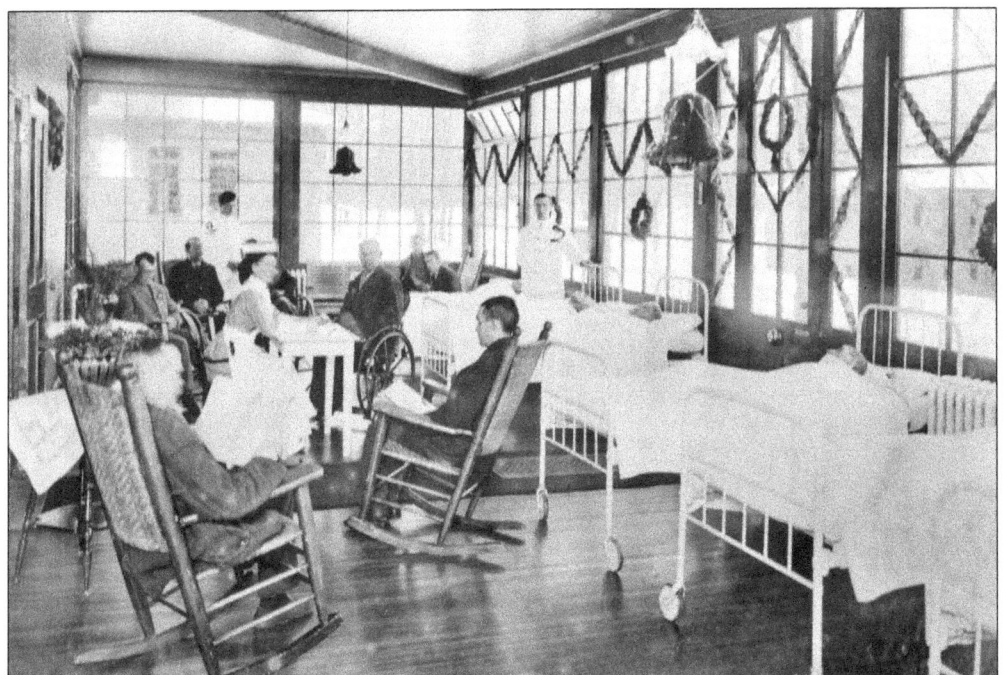

This image taken around the beginning of the 20th century shows a male ward at the Inwood building. Around the room, holiday decorations hang cheerfully, and snow covers the grounds out the windows. Beds were on wheels so that patients who could not walk could still enjoy the same social areas and views of the grounds other men had.

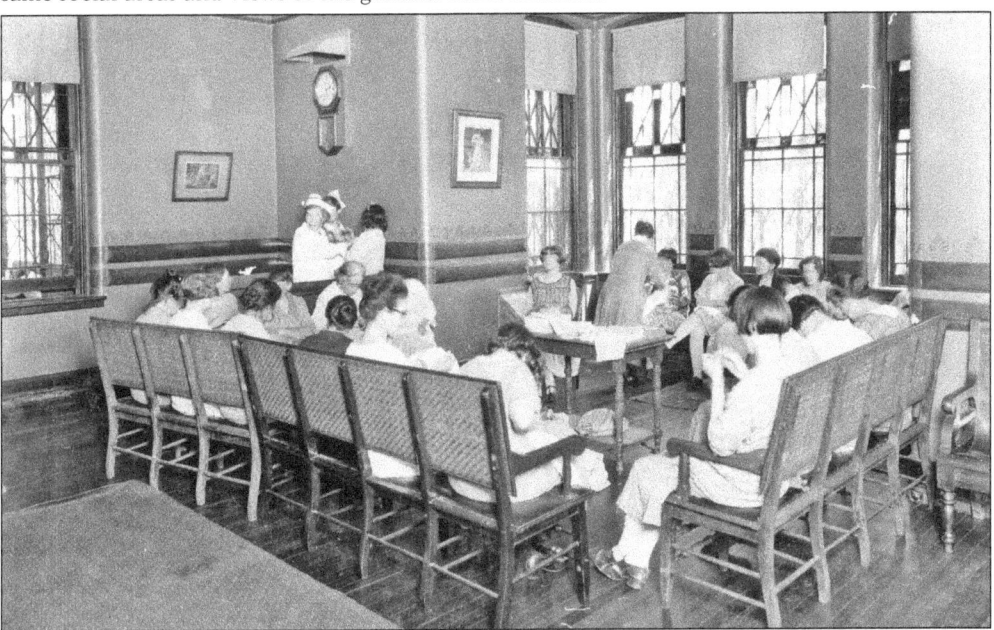

This image taken at the beginning of the 20th century in the north wing shows a typical afternoon crafts group in a day hall. Take notice of the items hung around the ward, a clock, paintings, and a small table—all items that could be found in an average living room. Items were not unnecessarily restricted on wards for low-risk patients.

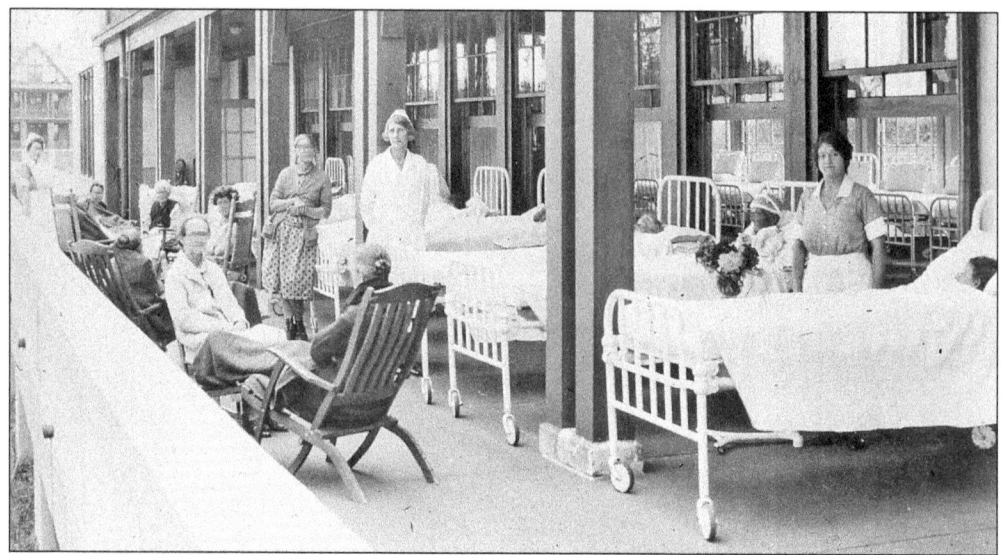

Lakeview was utilized as a tuberculosis quarantine and treatment hospital building. This 1920s image shows patients resting on the porch. Fresh-cut flowers from the hospital greenhouse sit in vases. Note the number of windows in the building, which is almost entirely glass. This is to allow a large amount of airflow to limit spread of tuberculosis through contaminated air. The windows have no security features to keep anyone in, not an obvious thought when one thinks of a psychiatric hospital.

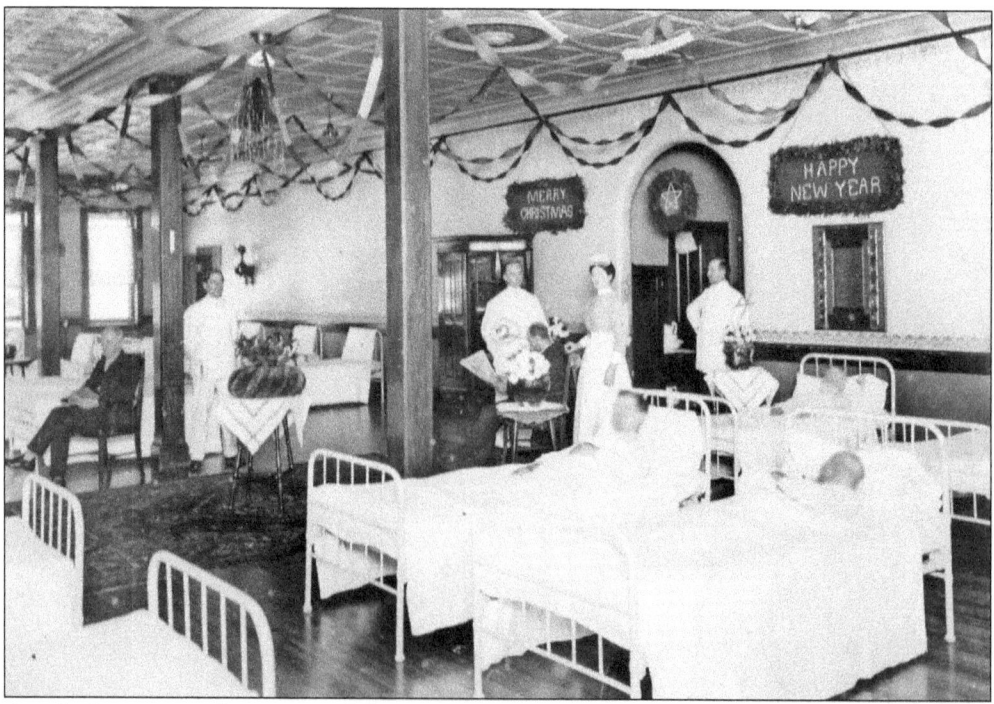

A male dormitory is shown around the turn of the 20th century. It is undoubtedly Christmastime, as signs wish all a merry season. Highlighting holidays was not only important for obvious social reasons, it allowed the continuity of the outside world's calendar while patients were hospitalized. This helped create a feeling of connection and even family spirt at Hudson River.

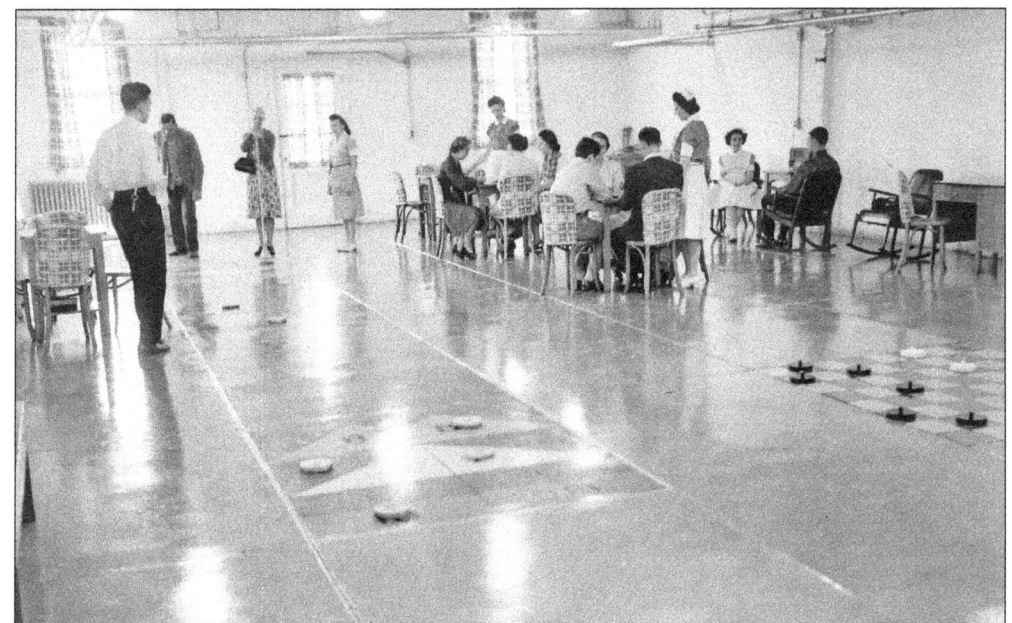

Not all patients were able to live in unlocked buildings or attend recreation in unsecured spaces. Above, a recreation room on the ground floor of Ryon Hall shows a secure space for leisure. Below, a man and women play an oversized game of checkers on the floor. To the left, an attendant watches over the area. The same recreation room is shown in 1951. Shuffleboard was another popular game played by patients at the hospital. Some wards had shuffleboard courts painted down long hallways. Above, a male and female enjoy a game while others play cards and Ping-Pong.

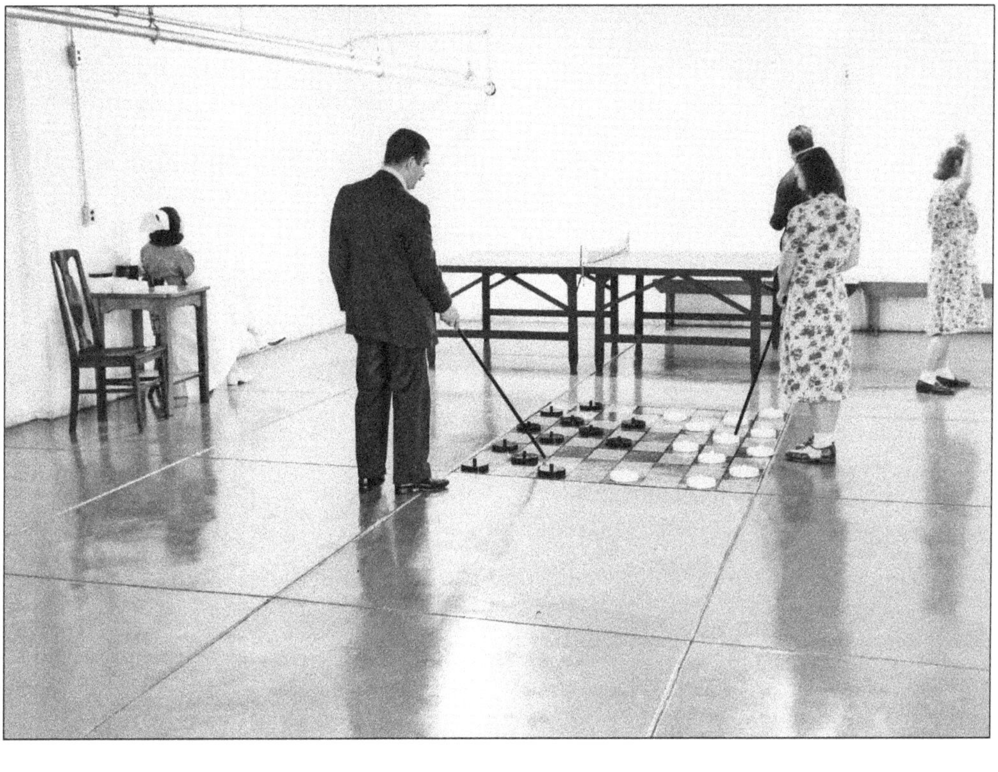

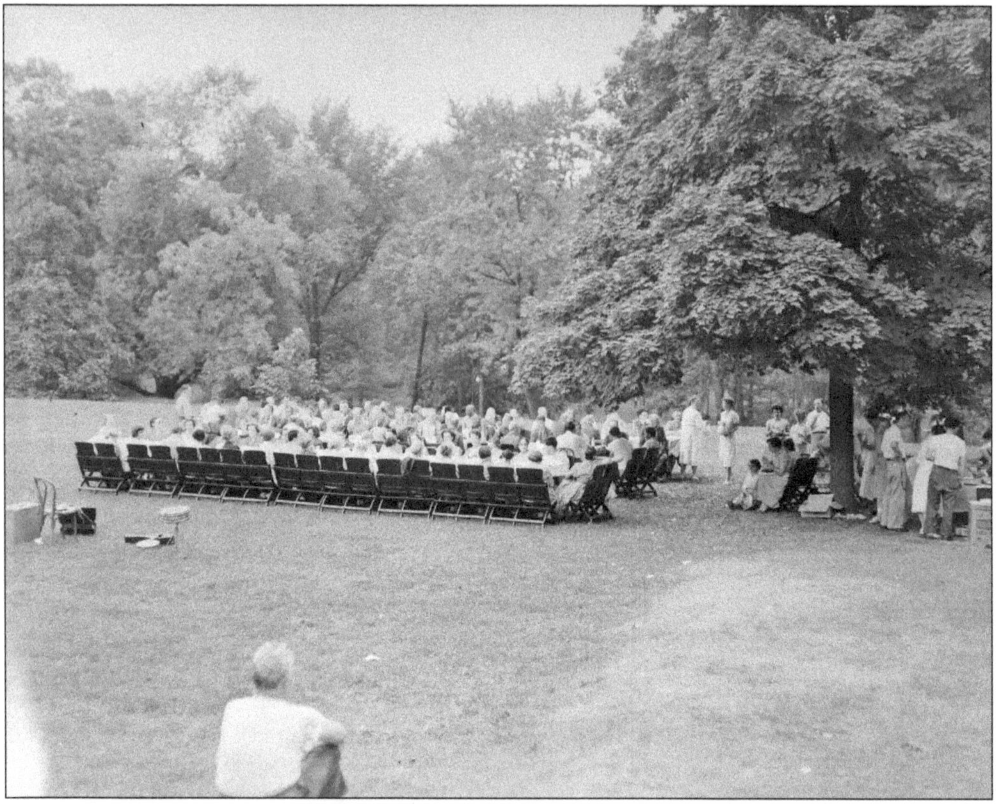

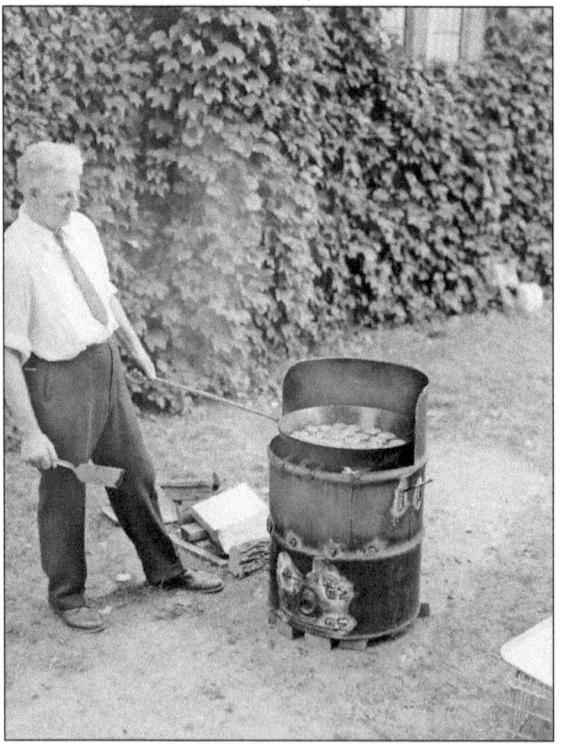

Barbecues were common, weather permitting. Ward staff would aid the kitchen staff in grilling and serving food outside. Eating communal meals together was a time for staff and patients to forget, in a sense, where they were and often bond over the experience. Almost all patients at the hospital had an opportunity to engage in this activity. This particular picnic took place in the summer of 1952 outside Avery Chapel. Patients and staff from the north and south wings enjoyed this event together.

Physical activity was thought to be paramount for good mental health at Hudson River many years before the general public caught on to this fact. Not all activity was in the form of organized sports. Here at a field day in 1952 are two such examples of team sports. Below, a barrel roll competition for young men takes place. At right, a good old-fashioned potato sack race is run on the same day. This was a great opportunity for patients to make friends over fond memories instead of bonding only over tragedies in their lives, as often was the case. After the activities this day, a clam bake for all the participants followed down at the boathouse.

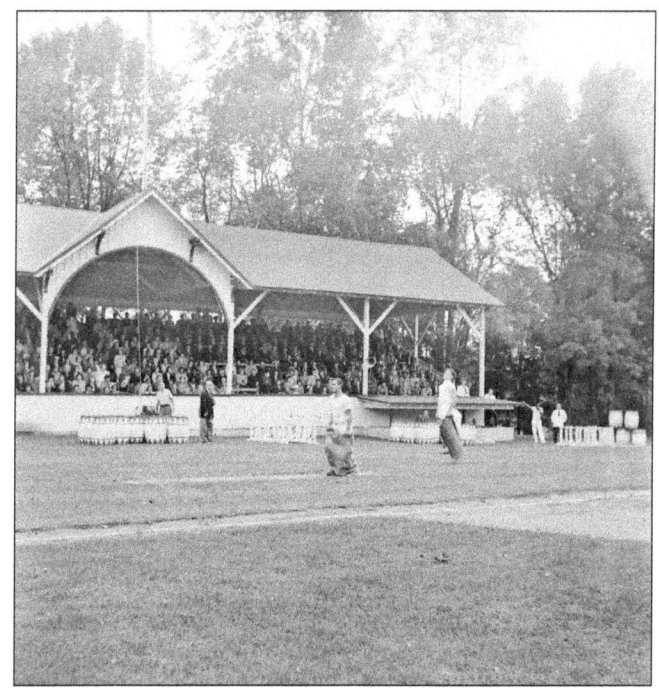

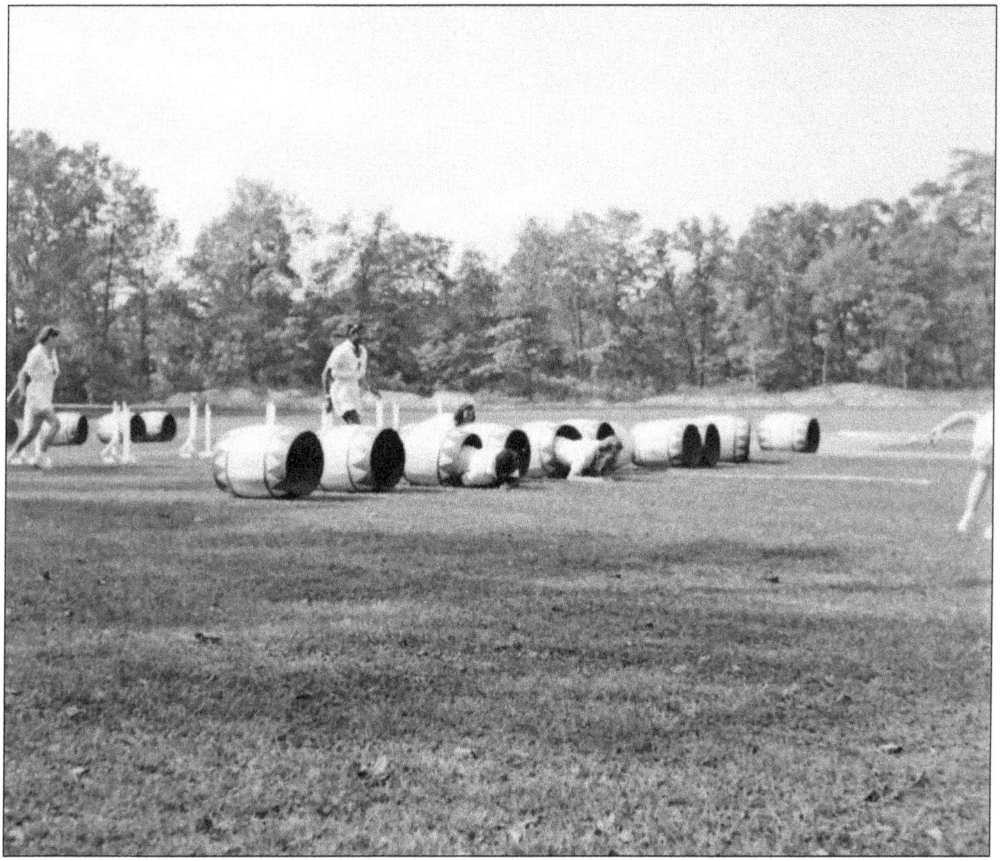

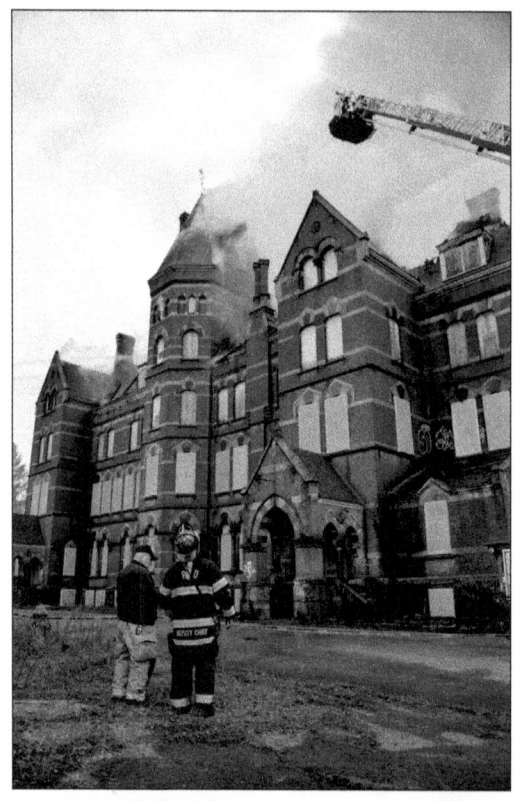

These two images were taken at the scene of a recent and tragic fire at Hudson River's old main building. The photograph at left shows firemen looking on as smoke bellows out of the eaves of the main building during the April 27, 2018, fire that broke out before dawn on the property. Below, an aerial image shows the damage to the South Wing (right) that occurred in the spring of 2007; the recent damage to the administration building (center) leaves the building a shell of its former grand self. This tragic event leaves the future preservation and reuse of this once grand structure uncertain. The authors of this book, former staff, and community members alike grieve the loss as a wincing reminder of a once bustling and robust facility left shuttered. (Left, Battalion 6 Photography; below, Phillip Gazard.)

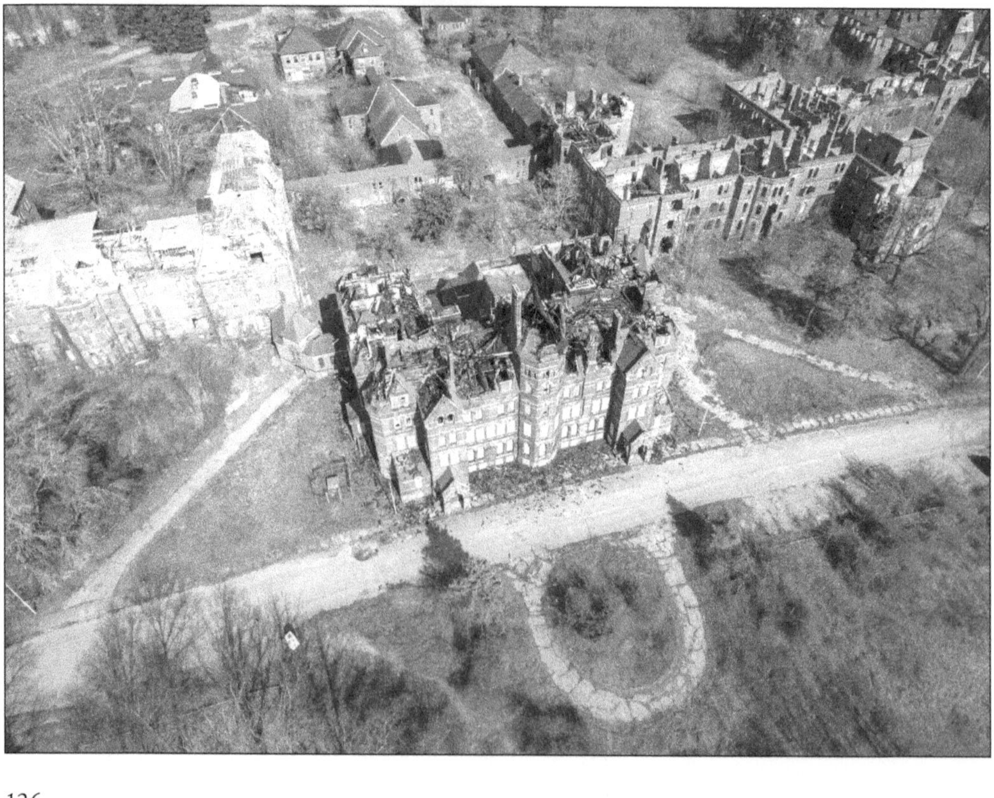

About the Hudson River State Hospital Nurses Alumni Association

Founded in 1934, the Hudson River State Hospital Nurses Alumni Association continues to promote the advancement of mental health and its allied areas by making financial contributions to local mental health associations. The alumni association works to advance the standards of the registered professional nurse and nursing by providing for a yearly scholarship award to an enrolled student in the nursing program at Dutchess Community College. The association promotes good fellowship among members by planning and holding meetings and social activities of interest. Additionally, the Hudson River State Hospital Nurses Alumni Association continues to preserve the rich cultural history of public mental health where the majority of its members were trained and employed. All members are volunteers dedicated to progressing the future of nursing, as well as mental health, by objectively presenting the past of psychiatric care to contemporary citizens, professionals, and students.

Visit us at
arcadiapublishing.com

www.ingramcontent.com/pod-product-compliance
Lightning Source LLC
Chambersburg PA
CBHW060922170426
43191CB00025B/2459